ANXIETY IN RELATIONSHIP

A ROADMAP

11 PRVEN TECHIQUES

Turn Insecurity, Jealousy, and Attachment into a Gift and
Break the Negative Thought Spirals Preventing You from
Nurturing Life-Long Bonds

A. MARIE SMITH

First Printing Edition, 2021
Printed in the United States of America
Available from Amazon.com and other retail outlet

TABLE OF CONTENTS

INTRODUCTION   7

PART ONE: BLACK AND WHITE THEORY   10

CHAPTER 1: ANXIETY AND RELATIONSHIP   11
What Causes Relationship Anxiety?   14
Understanding and Overcoming Relationship Anxiety   16
How does Relationship Anxiety Affect Us?   16
How Anxiety Can Affect Your Sex Life   17
Insecurity   19
Relationship Insecurity   20
Anxiety Interferes with Everyday Life   22

CHAPTER 2: STYLES OF ATTACHMENT   25
The 4 Attachment Styles   28
Attachment Questionary   32

CHAPTER 3: FEAR OF ABANDONMENT   37
Types of Fear of Abandonment   38
Symptoms of Fear of Abandonment   39
Disorders   40
Examples of Fear of Abandonment   41
Healing Abandonment Issues   42
Getting-to-Know-One-Another   43
About Your Partner Worksheet   45
Coping Strategies   47
Jealousy   48
How to Stop Jealousy   58
Wrapping Up   59

PART TWO: JUMP-OFF YOUR HEALING AND DEEPEN YOUR RELATIONSHIP 61

CHAPTER 4: TIME TO STOP STEALING THE MAGIC 62

TECHNIQUE 1: CHANGING YOURSELF TO REDUCE TOXICITY IN YOUR RELATIONSHIP 64
Visualization 65
What is the Meaning of Neuroplasticity? 71
The Theory and Principles of Neuroplasticity 72
What is Cognitive Behaviour Therapy? 73
Your Higher Self 75
8 Ways to Develop a More Positive Attitude 77
Understanding the Underlying Issues in Your Relationship 82

TECHNIQUE 2: CULTIVATE SELF-COMPASSION 83
An Introduction to Self-Compassion 83
5 Ways to Practice Self-Compassion 84
Why Self-Care? 88

TECHNIQUE 3: DEVELOP SELF-AWARENESS 92
4 Proven Benefits of Self-Awareness 93
Examples of Self-Awareness Skill 94
3 Ways to Cultivate Self-Awareness 96
Body Language 97
Emotions 104
5 Steps for Improving your Emotional Intelligence 105
How to Use Emotions to Your Advantage 110

TECHNIQUE 4: INCREASE LOW SELF-ESTEEM 112
Understanding Self-Esteem 112
7 Ways to Improve Your Self-Esteem 114

CHAPTER 5: LIGHT UP YOUR RELATIONSHIP 117

TECHNIQUE 5: OVERCOMING OBSTACLES IN YOUR RELATIONSHIP TO EASE ANXIETY 117
The 36 Questions 119
Keys to Communicating in Relationships 123
Deceit vs. Lying 129
Understanding The Reasons For Deceitful Behavior 129
The Warning Signs 131
Painful Events or Occurrences in Life 132
How to Solve the Main 5 Relationship Problems 138
Things to Do to Minimize Marriage Problems 142
7 Ways to Be More Open to New Experiences 142

TECHNIQUE 6: CREATING A SENSE OF SECURITY IN YOUR RELATIONSHIP **144**
Root Causes of Insecurity 144
Types of Insecurities 146
How Insecurity Can Ruin a Relationship 147
Five Ways to Increase Security in Your Relationship 148
How to Help your Partner Feel More Secure 149

TECHNIQUE 7: COMMUNICATION IS THE KEY TO A HAPPY RELATIONSHIP **150**
Communicating Clearly in a Relationship 150
Listening and Communication 152
Improving Communication in a Relationship 152
5 Tips for Communicating Better in Your Relationship 154

TECHNIQUE 8: KEEP YOUR RELATIONSHIP FLOURISHING **157**
7 Way to Keep Your Relationship Alive 159

TECHNIQUE 9: RESOLVING YOUR DIFFERENCES **166**
Check Your Focus 167
Talk To One Another 168
Make Opportunity Out Of Conflict 168
Ask Appropriate Questions 169
Practice Forgiveness 169

CHAPTER 6: LONGING FOR CONNECTIONS **171**

TECHNIQUE 10: MAKE NEW FRIENDS **173**
What to Look for in a Friend? 174
How to Make new Friends: Where to Start 176

TECHNIQUE 11: GET SUPPORT FROM YOUR OTHER-HALF **179**
5 Ways to Cope With It 181
How to Support Your Partner 184
The Easiest Ways To Be a More Supportive Partner 189

CONCLUSION **190**

THANK YOU **193**

INTRODUCTION

Whether single or in a relationship, many people believe that they'll never be happy in love. They feel lonely and want companionship— not just a buddy to sit next to at a movie, but a friend, confidante, and lover to accompany them through that greatest of all adventures we call life. They often fear that their partners will bolt once they get to know "the real me". Sometimes they feel that their partners appreciate the things they do. But this isn't enough. After all, what if their performance falters? Then there's the ever-present concern of whether anyone would truly be there fo them if they let themselves be vulnerable by looking to that person for support, comfort, and reassurance.

If you relate to any of these struggles, then this book is for you. I suffered from anxiety which made my loving relationship very miserable. I spend years reading, researching, doing coaching sections and therapy and soon until I managed to overcome my fears and limitations. Now I am on a happy long-term relationship for several years and finally able to live the fairy tale I always had in the mind. Inspired by the results of friends I already supported, I decided to put everything I learnt, the techniques and exercises that helped me the most together in this book hoping to positively impact the reader life as well.

During the early months and years of your life, you developed a certain style of connecting with—and attaching to—others.

Though you may not have been aware of this until adolescence or adulthood (or maybe it's still unclear), your current style is probably fundamentally the same as what was nurtured in childhood. If your early experiences left you questioning your sense of being worthy of love, fearful of being rejected, or with an unquenchable thirst for reassurance, then you probably still feel this way. It could also be that painful experiences later in life intensified anxiety about relationships that previously lurked under the surface. But the basic vulnerability to this attachment-related anxiety probably developed in childhood. It's important to understand that attachment-related anxiety does not have to be in response to any obviously abusive or harmful parenting; in fact, it most often is not. Many people with attachment related anxiety come from very lovings homes. Unfortunately, their parents' own struggles or difficult or traumatic circumstances interfered with

One crucial element in nurturing personal growth is developing greater self-awareness.

This includes being aware of your thoughts, acknowledging and consciously experiencing your emotions, and understanding what makes you tick. These tasks can be difficult, especially when you are facing unpleasant or conflicting aspects of yourself. However, they give you a better appreciation for your struggles. Such self-awareness frequently helps people feel a greater sense of well-being and, by itself, often facilitates change—such as reducing attachment-related anxiety and nurturing healthier relationships. As important as self-awareness is, it's equally important to recognize that it occurs in the context of your relationship with yourself. And many people are too hard on themselves. Just as you would attend to a hurt child by being nurturing, it is extremely helpful to approach yourself in a compassionate manner.

This guide explains, in easy-to- understand language, how your relationship struggles first formed; what about this process makes change so hard; and how those difficulties can be overcome so that you can enjoy a secure, lasting love.

While the main thrust of this book is to help you understand what you can do to find happiness in an intimate relationship, the ideas that I present can also help you to understand your partner better. Sometimes a window into your partner's world is exactly what you need to relate to him or her more compassionately, which in turn can help you to nurture a healthier relationship.

Make notes in the margins. Re-read sections as necessary, perhaps even pausing in a given section to work on applying it to your life before moving on. Also, give yourself time to engage with the exercises, rather than just trying to "get them done." I strongly suggest that you keep a journal to respond to the exercises, expand on your insights, and reflect on them later. Because the chapters build on each other, I sometimes refer to exercises in previ   completing new ones.

PART ONE: BLACK AND WHITE THEORY

CHAPTER 1: ANXIETY AND RELATIONSHIP

Relationships can be one of the most pleasurable things on the planet... but they can also be a breeding ground for anxious thoughts and feelings. Relationship anxieties can arise at pretty much any stage of courtship. For many single people, just the thought of being in a relationship can stir up stress. If and when people do start dating, the early stages can present them with endless worries:

"Does he/she truly likes me?"

"Will this work out?"

"How serious is this?"

Unfortunately, these worries don't tend to subside in the later stages of a romantic union. In fact, as things get closer between a couple, anxiety can get even more intense. Thoughts come flooding in like: "Can this last?"

"Do I really like him/her?" "Should we slow down?" "Am I really ready for this kind of commitment?" "Is he/she losing interest?"

All this worrying about our relationships can make us feel pretty alone. It can lead us to create distance between ourselves and our partner. At its worst, anxiety can push us to give upon love altogether. Learning more about the causes and effects of relationship anxiety can help us to identify the negative thinking and actions that can sabotage our love lives. How can we keep our anxiety in check and allow ourselves to be vulnerable to someone we love?

WHAT CAUSES RELATIONSHIP ANXIETY?

Put simply, falling in love challenges us in numerous ways we don't expect. The more we value someone else, the more we stand to lose. On many levels, both conscious and unconscious we become scared of being hurt. To a certain degree, we all possess a fear of intimacy. Ironically, this fear often arises when we are getting exactly what we want and when we're experiencing love as we never have or being treated in ways that are unfamiliar.

As we get into a relationship, it isn't just the things that go on between us and our partner that make us anxious,its the things we tell ourselves about what's going on. The "critical inner voice" is a term used to describe the mean coach we all have in our heads that criticizes us, feeds us bad advice and fuels our fear of intimacy. Its the one that tells us:

- "You're too ugly/fat/boring to keep his/her interest."
- "You'll never meet anyone, so why even try?"
- "You can't trust him. He's looking for someone better."
- "She doesn't really love you. Get out before you get hurt."

This critical inner voice makes us turn against ourselves and the people close to us. It can promote hostile, paranoid, and suspicious thinking that lowers our self-esteem and drives unhealthy levels of distrust, defensiveness, jealousy and anxiety. Basically, it feeds us a consistent stream of thoughts that undermine our happiness and make us worry about our relationship, rather than just enjoying it.

When we get in our heads, focusing on these worried thoughts, we become incredibly distracted from real relating with our partner. We may start to act out in destructive ways, making nasty comments or becoming childish or parental toward our significant other. For example, imagine your partner stays at work late one night. Sitting home alone, your inner critic starts telling you, "Where is she? Can you really believe her? She probably prefers being away from you. She's trying to avoid you. She doesn't even love you anymore." These thoughts can snowball in your mind until, the time your partner gets home, you're feeling insecure, furious or paranoid. You may act angry or cold, which then sets your partner off to feel frustrated and defensive. Pretty soon, you've completely shifted the dynamic between you. Instead of enjoying the time you have together, you may waste an entire night feeling withdrawn and upset with each other. You've now effectively forced the distance you initially feared. The culprit behind this self-fulfilling prophecy isn't the situation itself. It's that critical inner voice that colored your thinking, distorted your perceptions, and ultimately, led you down a destructive path.

When it comes to all of the things, we worry ourselves about in relationships, we are much more resilient than we think. In truth, we can handle the hurts and rejections that we so fear. We can experience pain, and eventually, heal. However, our critical inner voice tends to terrorize and catastrophize reality. It can rouse serious spells of anxiety about dynamics that don't exist and threats that aren't even tangible. Even when there are real things going on, someone breaksup with us or feels an interest in someone else, our critical inner voice will tear us apart in ways we don't deserve. It will completely distort reality and undermine our own strength and resilience. It's that cynical roommate that always gives bad advice. "You can't survive this. Just put your guard up and never be vulnerable to anyone else."

The defenses we form and critical voices we hear are based on our own unique experiences and adaptations. When we feel anxious or insecure, some of us have a tendency to become clingy and desperate in our actions and we may feel possessive or controlling toward our partner in response. Conversely, some of us will feel easily intruded on in our relationships. We may retreat from our partners, detach from our feelings of desire. We may react by being distant or guarded. These patterns of relating can come from our early attachment styles. Our attachment pattern is established in our childhood attachments and continue functioning as a working model for relationships in adulthood. It influences how each of us reacts to our needs and how we go about getting them met. Different attachment styles can lead us to experience different levels of relationship anxiety. You can learn more about what your attachment style is and how it impacts your romantic relationships here.

UNDERSTANDING AND OVERCOMING RELATIONSHIP ANXIETY

The specific critical inner voices we have about ourselves, our partner and relationships are formed out of early attitudes we were exposed to in our family or in society at large. Sexual stereotypes as well as attitudes that our influential caretakers had toward each other can infiltrate our point of view and shade our current perceptions. While, everyone's inner critic is different, some common critical inner voices include:

HOW DOES RELATIONSHIP ANXIETY AFFECT US?

As we shed light into our past, we quickly realize there are many early influences that have shaped our attachment pattern, our psychological defenses and our critical inner voice. All these factors contribute to our relationship anxiety and can lead us to sabotage our love lives in many ways. Listening to our inner critic and giving in to this anxiety can result in the following actions:

Cling – When we feel anxious, our tendency may be to act desperate toward our partner. We may stop feeling like the independent, strong people we were when we entered the relationship. As a result, we may find ourselves falling apart easily, acting jealous or insecure or no longer engaging in independent activities.

Control – When we feel threatened, we may attempt to dominate or control our partner. We may set rules about what they can and can't do just to all eviate our own feelings of insecurity or anxiousness. This behavior can alienate our partner and breed resentment.

Reject – If we feel worried about our relationship, one defense we may turn to is aloofness. We may become cold or rejecting to protect ourselves or to beat our partner to the punch. These actions can be subtle or overt, yet it is almost always a sure way to force distance or to stir up insecurity in our partner.

Withhold – Sometimes, as opposed to explicit rejection, we tend to withhold from our partner when we feel anxious or afraid. Perhaps things have gotten close, and we feel stirred up, so we retreat. We hold back little affections or give up on some aspect of our relationship altogether. Withholding may seem like a passive act, but it is one of the quietest killers of passion and attraction in a relationship.

Punish – Sometimes, our response to our anxiety is more aggressive, and we actually punish, taking our feelings out on our partner. We may yell and scream or give our partner the cold shoulder. It's important to pay attention to how much our actions are a response to our partner and how much are they a response to our critical inner voice.

Retreat – When we feel scared in a relationship, we may give up real acts of love and intimacy and retreat into a "fantasy bond." A fantasy bond is an illusion of connection that replaces real acts of love. In this state of fantasy, we focus on form over substance. We may stay in the relationship to feel secure but give up on the vital parts of relating. In a fantasy bond, we often engage in many of the destructive behaviors mentioned above as a means to create distance and defend ourselves against the anxiety that naturally comes with feeling free and in love. Learn more about the fantasy bond here.

HOW ANXIETY CAN AFFECT YOUR SEX LIFE

Most of the issues anxiety can cause in the bedroom can be worked through, especially with the help of a therapist. But first you have to recognize just how the emotions it brings on are sapping your sex life. You can overcome anxiety by distracting yourself, being open to your partner, and getting intimate in other ways without sexual intercourse. Sex should be fun, pleasurable, and stress-relieving. If it's not, read onto see how anxiety could be playing a role.

Anxiety Can Lower Your Libido

Anxious feelings can sink your sex drive in a number of ways. That overwhelmed feeling you get when anxiety kicks in can rail road sexy thoughts out of your brain, preventing you from being in the mood even if you were raring to go earlier in the day.

Panic and worry also have a physical effect on your body, ramping up the production of stress hormones like adrenaline that make you feel on edge. When your body can't physically relax, reveling in sexual sensations and getting close to a big O is going to be a lot more difficult.

And then there's the libido-lowering side effect of certain medications used to treat anxiety the drugs which help keep the condition from getting worse also tend to decrease your interest in getting it on.

It Keeps You from Being Body Confident

Getting naked in front of someone for the first time is nerve-racking for everyone. But when you have anxiety, you're more likely to feel intensely self-conscious, and you're more apt to obsess about so-called body flaws. "Women can be self-conscious about their body shape in general, or about a particular part, like their breasts, or about the way they smell, taste or perhaps move," says Steinberg. When you have anxiety, that self-consciousness is heightened.

"If women are continually being self-critical of themselves due to body shame, they shut down the ability to receive sexual pleasure fully and are unable to be fully present emotionally and physically during sexual scenarios," says Sari Cooper, director of Center for Love and Sex in New York City.

Anxiety Holds You Back from Intimacy

When you're seized by fear and panic, you may not want to be physically or emotionally close to your partner. And for women who have anxiety from past trauma, sexual touching and sex itself can be scary. If a woman is triggered by past trauma, it can cause her whole body to go into shut down mode, unable to experience enough arousal to tip her over the edge to a climax. Without realizing it, you might avoid sex or any foreplay, and that can create a strain on your relationship.

It Can Keep You from Asking for What You Want

It's often difficult even for close partners to share their preferences and fantasies. But anxiety can increase that challenge. Thing is, being honest will only make your sex life better, and it can be a relief to get any bottled up feelings off your chest.

"Whatever you want in bed is 100% normal and okay, and you will have a better relationship when you feel that you can be completely transparent with a partner," says Steinberg. It's hard to process that, though, when adrenaline is coursing through your body and making you feel as if danger is ahead.

Anxiety Makes It more Difficult to Orgasm

Clenched muscles, shallow breathing, goosebumps—these and other physical symptoms of anxiety block you from letting go and reaching climax. The condition "can raise your 'orgasmic threshold,'" says Steinberg, which is another term for how long it takes or how much stimulation you need to reach orgasm.

It can also put the brakes on lubrication, make flexing and bending your body uncomfortable, and even trigger vaginismus, a disorder that makes your vaginal muscles so tense and contracted, penetration is impossible. These physical changes, coupled with anxious thoughts, can further mess with your awareness of physical sexual stimulation, says Cooper, which inhibits orgasm.

INSECURITY

Insecurity is a feeling of inadequacy (not being good enough) and uncertainty. It produces anxiety about your goals, relationships, and ability to handle certain situations.

Everybody deals with insecurity from time to time. It can appear in all areas of life and come from a variety of causes. It might stem from a traumatic event, patterns of previous experience, social conditioning (learning rules by observing others), or local environments such as school, work, orhome.

It can also stem from general instability. People who experience unpredictable upsets in daily life are more likely to feel insecure about ordinary resources and routines.

Types of Insecurity

There are almost limitless areas of potential insecurity. Moreover, insecurity often bleeds over from one area of life into another. However, there are some types of insecurity that appear frequently, but I'm going to talk about only relationship insecurities since it would be of significant influence.

RELATIONSHIP INSECURITY

One of the most common kinds of insecurity concerns relationships or "attachments."

Attachment theory originated out of a desire to connect the attachment patterns of early childhood to later relationship patterns and expectations. When a child's "attachment figures," often parents or guardians, aren't reliably available and supportive, the child often feels insecure, forms a negative self-image and relationship models, and experiences greater emotional distress and maladjustment later in life.

Relationship or attachment insecurities don't need to begin in early childhood. They can arise wherever previous experience or personal insecurity undermines someone's security in their closest relationships.

Your gut instincts are those nagging feelings that alert you to potentially dangerous situations, or let you know when something may go wrong. These feelings are what keep you safe in dark parking garages, and what steer you towards good choices. But the problem is, it can often be difficult to tell the difference between intuition and anxiety.

When you are prone to anxiety, both mental and physical, the problem is that you really can't 'trust your gut,'" Melissa Weinberg, LCPC, psycho therapist and owner of Open Lines Counseling. "The difference between anxiety symptoms and gut reactions becomes very blurry." And symptoms can feel one in the same.

What feels like intuition — a thought that won't go away, butterflies in your stomach, etc. — might actually beanxiety. And vice versa. "If you struggle with anxiety, your gut is overactive and often interpreting benign external information, internal sensations, or passing thoughts as threats," Weinberg says. But the good thing is, it ispossible to wade through the murky waters and figure out what'swhat.

By talking with a therapist, for example, you can start to gather tools to better cope with anxiety, so it no longer gets in the way of your intuition. Here are a few things to keep in mind, so you can be better able to tell the difference.

Anxiety Doesn't Let Up

One of the easiest ways to tell the differencebetween a gut instinct and anxiety is by how long your symptoms last. "A gut instinct isoften a reaction to an immediate situation," Weinberg says. "Anxiety, on the other hand, might be present regardless of its relevance to your current experience."

Take that dark parking garage, for instance. If you experience a desire to run quickly to your car, that might be your gut instinct guiding you away from danger. But if you feel that level of anxiety all day long, well, it's probably anxiety.

Anxiety CausesYou to Worry About the Future

Anxiety tends to be future-focused in a very unhealthy way. So if "your head is swarming with hypotheticals and worst case scenarios," it's likely not your gut instinct.

Anxiety symptoms might even keep you up at night, asyou think ahead to work projects, worry about your health, or wonder about the future of your relationship. Unlike intuition, anxiety likes to zero in on things you can't control (AKA, the future).

Anxiety Causes Feelings of Uncertainty

While both anxiety and intuition can create an unsettled feeling, anxiety will likely lead to more uncertainty — while instincts will feel more concrete.

Your gut is your internal wisdom. You may be afraid to act on it but it feels certain, very much unlike anxiety which feels like uncertainty."

That's why, if you're waffling back and forth and can't decide what to do, you can rest assured whatever's on your mind is likely anxiety-fueled.

ANXIETY INTERFERES WITH EVERYDAY LIFE

Unlike gut instincts, anxiety doesn't have any redeeming qualities. And it may even start to negatively impact your life. So take note if you are starting to avoid certain situations, or can't seem to function in a healthy way.

When our 'intuition' or 'gut instinct' starts to interfere with how we're handling life, it can be an indication that we are struggling with anxiety.

A gut instinct may steer you away from an unsafe situation, but anxiety might steer you away from most situations. And when that's the case, you'll no longer be able to tell what's worth worrying about.

Anxiety Causes Many Prolonged Symptoms

It really can help to look at the actual definition of anxiety, in order to figure out what's causing your stressful feelings, especially if they're sticking around.

The DSM-V (the diagnostic manual mental health professionals use to diagnose disorders, including anxiety) outlines the specific symptoms of general anxiety, which include: excessive worry and anxiety, difficulty controlling the worry, and physical symptoms related to the anxiety, such as restlessness, fatigue, difficulty concentrating, irritability, muscle tension, and difficulty with sleep.

It maybe helpful to speak with a therapist, if you are experiencing these symptoms, since they can help you find ways to cope. Once you begin to heal yourself of anxiety, you'll be able to better tune into your intuition.

Gut Instincts Can Be Tested and Verified

One of the nice things about gut instincts is that they can be "easily tested," Weinberg says. "Anxious worry cannot." So if you want to tell which is which, look to your surroundings for some concrete evidence.

For example, if you have a 'gut instinct' that your basement is leaking during a storm, you can verify this easily with a visit to the basement," she says. If your basement is full ofwater, go ahead and thank your gut for tipping you off that something was wrong.

If, however, you are worried about the structure and safety of your house and can't stop thinking about when something might break or if the basement will flood next time it rains, these are doubts and uncertainties that fall under the umbrella of anxiety — not immediate danger. They are fueled by uncertainty and have no knowable answers.

Gut Instincts Are Based on Patterns

A gut instinct is how we feel 'right now.' It's based on a highly evolved project survival strategy based in pattern recognition. I stubbed my toe while walking in the kitchen. My gut instinct is that it might happen again. So now I amvery careful about my step placement moving forward.

Compare this to anxiety. "Anxiety would be if I projected that singular occurrence into a future-based fear of walking because now I feel it's not safe to walk,". See the difference?

Gut Instincts Help Center You

Gut instincts often cause everything to slow down, as they direct you where you need to go. "There is a center of calm knowing with gut instinct, a certainty on a specific topic," Reiki Master and intuitive Stephanie Whitehead, tells Bustle. This is very unlike anxiety, which tends to cause chaotic, scattered thinking.

Gut Instincts Often Have Solutions

When you have a gut instinct, it's often easy to solve whatever's bugging you: you can leave the dark parking garage, make a decision, or check your basement for flooding.

To go with the previous example, if it israining and youhave a feeling that your basement is flooding, you can do something about that. But, if you are awake in the middle of the night worrying about how to make necessary improvements to your house that might be a legitimate problem that impacts your life and needs a solution. But can you do something about it at 3 a.m.? Probably not. If something is truly wrong, there will bean immediate action that can be taken to address it. If the worry is not actionable, it is anxiety."

Even though it's not immediately fixable, you can certainly find ways to deal with anxiety by making healthy life style changes, speaking with a therapist, and possibly even taking medication. Once you are able to tone down anxiety symptoms, your gut instincts will be much clearer. And you'll have a much easier time telling the difference between the two.

CHAPTER 2: STYLES OF ATTACHMENT

The bond we form with our first primary caregiver, usually our parent. It's a universal human phenomenon that starts as early as in the womb, and the way we develop it eventually affects the way we find, keep, and end relationships. As already mentioned in the previous chapter, It's the theory that explains what kind of attachment we form in our adult relationships, particularly with our romantic partners.

Some relationships have compatible attachment styles, others are not so lucky. When you end up dating somebody with a different attachment style, it could lead to all kind of conflicts in the relationship. One of these conflicts could be about time. For example, attachment theory explains that some people expect to spend all of their free time with their partners while other people, however, neither want nor need to spend so much time with their partners. This difference can cause a struggle between two people as they try to agree on how much time to invest in the relationship.

Which Attachment Style Am I?

Have you seen the show *How I Met Your Mother?* It's about a bunch of flawed but lovable New Yorkers trying to find (or hang on to) love as they go through life's changes, which range from silly to momentous. It's a funny, feel good, and sometimes poignant sitcom but what I like most about it is that it's a perfect showcase of human attachment styles.

If you don't know what attachment styles are, or haven't ever seen the show, don't worry. Once you hear about the characters and how they personify each attachment style, you'll be sure to recognize yourself or people you know.

There are four major styles of attachment that people form early in life and generally tend to keep into adulthood. These styles are:

- Secure
- Dismissive-avoidant
- Anxious-preoccupied
- Fearful-avoidant (a.k.a., disorganized)

To figure out what style of attachment you tend to have, there are quizzes you can take (you can check out www.sapa-project.org, www.attachmentproject.com). They ask you to agree/disagree with statements like, "I easily develop emotional ties toothers," "If a partner pushes me to establish a commitment, I freak out inside," and, "If I'm not in a relationship, I am nobody." You can see that these items are probing the way we think of others and ourselves in the context of relationships and intimacy.

So what attachment style do you think you have? Well, let just see if you most closely relate to Ted, Barney, or someone else from *How I Met Your Mother*. This sitcom is about Ted recounting to his son, Luke, and daughter, Penny events that prompt him to meet their mother. In this first in a three-part series on attachment, we'll let the beloved HIMYM characters guide us through the four major attachment styles which are: secure attachment, anxious attachment, avoidant attachment and fearful attachment.

Attachment theory in psychology originates with the seminal work of John Bowlby (1958). In the 1930s, John Bowlby worked as a psychiatrist in a Child Guidance Clinic in London where he treated many emotionally disturbed children.

This experience led Bowlby to consider the importance of the child's relationship with their mother in terms of their social, emotional and cognitive development. Specifically, it shaped his belief about the link between early infant separations with the mother and later maladjustment, and led Bowlby to formulate his attachment theory.

Bowlby defined attachment as a 'lasting psychological connectedness between human beings.'

Bowlby (1958) proposed that attachment can be understood within an evolutionary context in that the caregiver provides safety and security for the infant. Attachment it is adaptive as it enhances the infant's chance of survival.

Your Parents Significantly Influence Attachment Style

I hate to say it, but your parents have a pretty big hand in how you relate to, pick, and connect with your romantic partners. This all started with a fascinating experiment done in the 1960's by John Bowlby and Mary Ainsworth. Bowlby and Ainsworth put children and parents through what's called the "Strange Situation" test.

The Strange Situation:

Imagine that as a child you were put into a big room. Your mom comes in. Your mom does not participate in your exploration of the room. A stranger comes in theroom, talks to your mom, and then approaches you. Your mom quietly exits the room.

How do you react?

Finally, your mom returns.

During this exercise, researchers are observing these behaviors:

How the child explores the room and plays with new toys throughout the experience.

What the child does when their parent disappears.

How the child reacts when alone with a stranger.

What the child does when the parent returns.

Based on how the child reacts, they were placed into four categories representing their attachment to their parent–these are the 4 attachment styles. Researchers believe you keep these attachment styles throughout your life and repeat them with partners, kids, and friends.

THE 4 ATTACHMENT STYLES

Dr. Phillip Shaver and Dr. Cindy Hazan took the parent-child research and applied it to romantic relationships. Here is an explanation of each style and what percentage of the population displays it.

1. Secure Attachment

Securely attached people tend to be less anxious and more satisfied with their relationships. The children who were securely attached were happy to explore and bring toys back to the parent. In other words, their parent was a kind of base they could explore around and come back to. Securely attached people have an easy time forming connections and have less doubt about the equality of the relationship. They also have an easier time reaching out for comfort.

2. Anxious Attachment

People who anxiously attach tend to worry more about their relationships. They are said to experience an 'emotional hunger' and are desperate for a fantasy type of love. Unlike, people with an anxious attachment tend to be desperate to form a fantasy bond of ideal love–even when this might not be possible or reciprocated. They tend to look for a partner who can rescue them or 'complete' them. Unfortunately, their desperation sometimes can push away the exact person they want closeness with. When they are afraid of losing their partner, they can become clingy, possessive, paranoid, or need constant attention.

3. Avoidant Attachment

Avoidant attachers tend to be emotionally distant from their partners. Avoidant attachers take pride in their independence and can see attachment as weakness. They like to process emotions on their own and don't like to share vulnerabilities with anyone else. Unfortunately, they tend to pull away when they need help most. They are not as attentive as their partners because they worry they will become too co-dependent, and this will take away their independence. They also can shut down emotionally during arguments or close themselves off from feelings.

4. Fearful Attachment

This also is called 'disoriented' or 'disorganized' attachment. These children seemed to volley between desperately needing their parent and pushing them away. People with this kind of attachment live in an ambivalent mindset where they swing from being afraid of connection to over-analyzing the equality or depth of their relationships. They tend to get overwhelmed easily and have unpredictable moods. At one moment they can smother their partner, and at the next they can disappear for a day or two without explanation.

You Are not Doomed to Your Attachment Style

Awareness is the first (and most important) step. What are your patterns? Do you tend to pull away or smother? Being honest with yourself and your partner is crucial. Second, it's important to treat your relationship as a foundation and develop it as a secure base. Researchers say people who change their attachment style are forming an "earned secure attachment." This means:

Avoiding rocky relationships: Frequent break-ups, fights, or rollercoaster emotions will destroy your chances at moving to a secure style.

Believing in growth: There is no such thing as a perfect relationship or perfect partner. The more we understand that we can grow into deeper and deeper love, the more energy we put into a relationship (instead of doubting it or dismissing it).

Seeking secure partners: If you are looking for your ideal partner, it is important to think about how they attach. Anxious and Avoidant attachers can seek out secure attachers to become more secure themselves.

The Secure Base

Your relationship can be a home base, a touch stone, a foundation for you. In the right relationship, you seek out a satisfying and loving mutual connection. I found this study on attachment styles particularly interesting: It's not that secure people don't need support, it's that they don't ask for it.

Changing Your Attachment Style is a Long and Difficult Process

You can definitely try to change your particular attachment style, but that's a reallyblong and difficult process. According to attachment theory, we develop our attachment style when weare small children. It's usually based on the relationship wehad with our parents.

Instead, we're going to talk about the different types of attachment styles and which combinations are better for relationships. If youcan identify your exact attachment style, you can find a partner who fits your needs. This, ofcourse, is the ideal situation. If you're already in a relationship, however, and your attachment combination isn't so good, don't worry! There's still hope for you and your significant other.

Each Attachment Combination has a Different Outlook for the Relationship

If either person has a secure attachment style, then the relationship has a positive outlook. Attachment theory tells us that the person with a secure attachment styleis able to validate their partner's concerns. They can even help their less secure partner overcome their insecurities.

The anxious + anxious combination is challenging. People with this attachment style are able to read small changes in emotion and behavior. This perceptive ability combined with their anxious insecurity results in jumping to conclusions. [1] In short, two insecure anxious people have the potential to experience a relationship full of drama, jealousy, and arguments. The same happens for the insecure disorganized + insecure disorganized combination.

When an avoidant one pairs up with another avoidant one, there'll be little communication, which may seem to be fine at the beginning as both aren't demanding. But as time goes by the connection will become weaker and it's hard to sustain the relationship.

Toxic Combination

If the two attachment styles are anxious and avoidant, things are going to be difficult. You should probably mentally prepare yourself for the kind of issues that this combination might bring to your life. If you're thinking about getting into this romance, think again.

Interestingly, these two types of attachment are often drawn together. That's because they almost complement each other. An anxious person has fear of losing their partner and so they wait for the avoidant person to decide to commit to the relationship. This combination validates the avoidant person's behavior.

As insecure disorganized style is a combination of the anxious type and the avoidant type, when the anxious side comes up, it'll be a disaster with the avoidant type. When the avoidant side comes up, conflicts will arise with the anxious type. That's why both insecure disorganized + insecure avoidant and insecure disorganized+ insecure anxious arenot likely to work.

Be Honest with Yourself to Identify your Attachment Style

In order to find someone who fits your attachment style, you must first identify it. Think about the way you react to the things your partner does.

If they tell you they'll call at 6:00 pm and they don't call until 6:30 pm, do you spend that half hour worrying what could have possibly gone wrong? Do you start feeling vulnerable or thinking you've probably been abandoned? Be honest with yourself, you've probably been known to pout or start arguments with your partner. Sound familiar? You're probably an insecure anxious type.

Think about how you feel after you spend a lot of time with your significant other. Do you need some time to yourself? Or maybe you feel like being in a longterm relationship means you'll lose your identity or independence. If this sounds like you, you could be have an insecure avoidant attachment type.

Observe Your Partner's Behavior to Find out Their Attachment Style

It may seem more difficult to identify your significant other's attachment style, but it's not impossible. You might not know exactly how they feel internally, but you can observe their behaviors. Think about how they react to your concerns. If you've had a bad day and you come home talking about it, what do they say? Do you feel ignored, like they just aren't interested? They might have an insecure avoidant attachment style.

What happens when you're running late to a date? If they start sending texts after only 3 minutes to ask if you're still coming, they might be an anxious type.

No relationship is perfect and certainly no relationship is bound to fail just because of attachment styles. By understanding your person attachment style and that of your partner's, though, you can make real progress toward ensuring your future happiness together.

ATTACHMENT QUESTIONARY

The first step toward applying attachment theory to your life is to get to know yourself and those around you from an attachment perspective. In the next chapter, we'll walk you through the process of determining your partner or prospective partner's attachment style based on various clues. But let's begin by assessing the person you know best—yourself.

Following is a questionnaire designed to measure your attachment style— the way you relate to others in the context of intimate relationships. This questionnaire is based on the Experience in Close Relationship (ECR) questionnaire.

Attachment styles are stable but plastic. Knowing your specific attachment profile will help you understand yourself better and guide you in your interactions with others. Ideally, this will result in more happiness in your relationships.

How to Answer the Questions:

Answer A, B, or C to each question.

A: 1-4, not really true
B: 5-7, fairly right
C: 8-10, extremely righ

If the answer is untrue, don't mark the item at all.

Questions:

1. *I often worry that my partner will stop loving me.*

2. *I find it easy to be affectionate with my partner.*

3. *I fear that once someone gets to know the real me, s/he won't like who I am.*

4. *I find that I bounce back quickly after a breakup. It's weird how I can just put someone out of my mind.*

5. *When I'm not involved in a relationship, I feel somewhat anxious and incomplete.*

6. *I find it difficult to support my partner when s/he is feeling down emotionally.*

7. *When my partner is away, I'm afraid that s/he might become interested in someone else.*

8. *I feel comfortable depending on romantic partners.*

9. *My independence is more important to me than my relationships.*

10. *I prefer not to share my innermost feelings with my partner.*

11. *When I show my partner how I feel, I'm afraid s/he will not feel the same about me.*

12. *I am generally satisfied with my romantic relationships.*

13. *I don't feel the need to act out much in my romantic relationships.*

14. *I think about my relationships a lot.*

15. *I find it difficult to depend on romantic partners.*

16. *I tend to get very quickly attached to a romantic partner.*

17. *I have little difficulty expressing my needs and wants to my partner.*

18. *I sometimes feel angry or annoyed with my partner without knowing why.*

19. *I am very sensitive to my partner's moods.*

20. *I believe most people are essentially honest and dependable.*

21. *I prefer casual sex with uncommitted partners to intimate sex with one person.*

22. *I'm comfortable sharing my personal thoughts and feelings with my partner.*

23. *I worry that if my partner leaves me, I might never find someone else.*

24. *It makes me nervous when my partner gets too close.*

25. *During a conflict, I tend to impulsively do or say things I later regret rather than be able to reason about things.*

26. *An argument with my partner doesn't usually cause me to question our entire relationship*

27. *My partners often want me to be more intimate than I feel comfortable being.*

28. *I worry that I'm not attractive enough.*

29. *Sometimes people see me as boring because I create little drama in relationships.*

30. *I miss my partner when we're apart, but then when we're together, I feel the need to escape.*

31. *When I disagree with someone, I feel comfortable expressing my opinions.*

32. *I hate feeling that other people depend on me.*

33. *If I notice that someone, I'm interested in is checking out other people, I don't let it faze me. I might feel a pang of jealousy, but it's fleeting.*

34. *If I notice that someone, I'm interested in is checking out other people, I feel relieved—it means s/he's not looking to make things exclusive.*

35. *If I notice that someone, I'm interested in is checking out other people, it makes me feel depressed.*

36. *If someone I've been dating begins to act cold and distant, I may wonder what's happened, but I'll know it's probably not about me.*

37. *If someone I've been dating begins to act cold and distant, I'll probably be indifferent; I might even be relieved.*

38. *If someone I've been dating begins to act cold and distant, I'll worry that I've done something wrong.*

39. *If my partner wants to break up with me, I will try my best to show her/him what she/he is missing (a little jealousy can't hurt).*

40. *If someone I've been dating for several months tells me she/he wants to stop seeing me, I'd feel hurt at first, but I'd get over it.*

41. *Sometimes when I get what I want in a relationship, I'm not sure what I want anymore.*

42. *I won't have much of a problem staying in touch with my ex (strictly platonic)—after all, we have a lot in common.*

Scoring Key

- Add up all your checked boxes in column A:
- Add up all your checked boxes in column B:
- Add up all your checked boxes in column C:

The more statements you check in a category, the more you will display the corresponding attachment style characteristics.

- Category A represents the anxious attachment style
- Category B represents the secure attachment style
- Category C represents the avoidant attachment style

Anxious - You love to be very close to your romantic partners and have the capacity for great intimacy. However, you often fear that your partner does not wish to be as close as you would like him/her to be. Relationships tend to consume a large part of your emotional energy. You tend to be very sensitive to small fluctuations in your partner's moods and actions, and although your senses are often accurate, you take your partner's behaviors too personally. You experience a lot of negative emotions within the relationship and get easily upset. As a result, you tend to act out and say things you later regret. If the other person provides a lot of security and reassurance, however, you are able to shed much of your preoccupation and feel contented.

Secure - Being warm and loving in a relationship comes naturally to you. You enjoy being intimate without becoming overly worried about your relationships. You take things in stride when it comes to romance and don't get easily upset over relationship matters. You effectively communicate your needs and feelings to your partner and are strong at reading your partner's emotional cues and responding to them. You share your successes and problems with your mate, and are able to be there for him or her in times of need.

Avoidant - It is very important for you to maintain your independence and self-sufficiency, and you often prefer autonomy to intimate relationships. Even though you do want to be close to others, you feel uncomfortable with too much closeness and tend to keep your partner at arm's length. You don't spend much time worrying about your romantic relationships or about being rejected. You tend not to open up to your partners, and they often complain that you are emotionally distant. In relationships, you are often on high alert for any signs of control or impingement on your territory by your partner.

CHAPTER 3: FEAR OF ABANDONMENT

Fear of abandonment is the overwhelming worry that people close to you will leave.

Anyone can develop a fear of abandonment. It can be deeply rooted in a traumatic experience you had as a child or a distressing relationship in adulthood.

If you fear abandonment, it can be almost impossible tomaintain healthy relationships. This paralyzing fear can lead you to wall yourself off to avoid getting hurt. Or you might be inadvertently sabotaging relationships.

The first step in overcoming your fear is to acknowledge why you feel this way. You may be able to address your fears on your own or with therapy. But fear of abandonment may also be part of a personality disorder that needs treatment.

TYPES OF FEAR OF ABANDONMENT

You may fear that someone you love is going to physically leave and not come back. You may fear that someone will abandon your emotional needs. Either can hold you back in relationships with a parent, partner, or friend. The types of fear of abandonment include: fear of emotional abandonment, fear of abandonment in children, abandonment anxiety in relationships.

1. Fear of Emotional Abandonment

It may be less obvious than physical abandonment, but it is no less traumatic.

We all have emotional needs. When those needs aren't met, you may feel unappreciated, unloved, and disconnected. You can feel very much alone, even when you're in a relationship with someone who's physically present.

If you've experienced emotional abandonment in the past, especially as a child, you may live in perpetual fear that it will happen again.

2. Fear of Abandonment of Children

Young ones, especially toddlers, go through a separate anxiety stage. They might cry, scream or even refuse when their guardian has to leave. At this period, children find it difficult to grasp when or if they will return. When kids now start to realize that their loved ones do come back, they outweigh their fear.

3. Abandonment Anxiety in Relationships

You may be afraid to let yourself be vulnerable in a relationship. You may have trust issues and worry excessively about your relationship. That can make you suspicious of your partner.

In time, your anxieties can cause the other people to pull back, perpetuating the cycle.

SYMPTOMS OF FEAR OF ABANDONMENT

If you fear abandonment, you might recognize some ofthesesymptomsand signs:

- Overly sensitiveto criticism
- Difficulty trusting in others
- Difficulty making friends unless you can be sure they like you
- Taking extreme measures to avoid rejection or separation
- Pattern of unhealthy relationships
- Getting attached to people too quickly, then moving on just as quickly
- Difficulty committing to a relationship
- Working too hard to please the other person
- Blaming yourself when things don't workout
- Staying in a relationship even if it's not healthy for you

Abandonment Issues in Relationships

If you fear abandonment in your current relationship, it may be due to having been physically or emotionally abandoned in the past. For example:

As a child, you may have experienced the death or desertion of a parent or caregiver.

- You may have experienced parental neglect
- You may have been rejected by your parents
- You went through a prolonged illness of a loved one
- A romantic partner may have left you suddenly or behaved in an untrustworthy manner
- Such events can lead to a fear of abandonment

DISORDERS

Avoidant PersonalityDisorder

Avoidant personality disorder is a personality disorder that can involve fear of abandonment resulting in the person feeling socially inhibitedor inadequate. Some other signs and symptoms are:

- Nervousness
- Poor self-esteem
- Intense fear of being negatively judged or rejected
- Discomfort in social situations
- Avoidance of group activities and self-imposed social isolation

Borderline Personality Disorder

Borderline personality disorderis another personality disorder in which intense fearof abandonment canplay a role. Other signs and symptoms can include:

- Unstable relationships
- Distorted self-image
- Extreme impulsiveness
- Moodswings and inappropriate anger
- Difficulty being alone

Many people who have borderline personality disorder say they were sexually or physically abused as children. Others grew up amid intense conflict or had family members with the same condition.

Separation Anxiety Disorder

If a child doesn't outgrow separation anxiety and it interferes with daily activities, they may have separation anxiety disorder.

Other signs and symptoms of separation anxiety disorder can include frequent:

- Panic attacks
- Distress at the thought of being separated from loved ones

- Refusal to leave home without a loved one or be left home alone
- Nightmares involving being separated from loved ones
- Physical issues, like stomachache or headache, when separated from loved ones

Teens and adults can have separation anxiety disorder too.

Long-Term Effects of Fear of Abandonment

Long-term effects of fear of abandonment can include:

- Difficult relationships with peers and romantic partners
- Low self-esteem
- Trust issues
- Anger issues
- Mood swings
- Codependency
- Fear of intimacy
- Anxiety disorders
- Panic disorders
- Depression

EXAMPLES OF FEAR OF ABANDONMENT

Here are a few examples of what fear of abandonment can look like:

- Your fear is so significant that you don't allow yourself to get close enough to anyone to let that happen. You may think, "No attachment, no abandonment."
- You worry obsessively about your perceived faults and what others may think of you.
- You're the ultimate people pleaser. You don't want to take any chances that someone won't like you enough to stick around.
- You're absolutely crushed when someone offers a bit of criticism or gets upset with you in anyway.
- You overreact when you feel slighted.
- You feel inadequate and unappealing.

- You breakup with a romantic partner so they can't break up with you.
- You're clingy even when the other person asks for space.
- You're often jealous, suspicious, orcritical of your partner.

Diagnosing Fear of Abandonment

Fear of abandonment isn't a diagnosable mental health disorder, but it cancertainly be identified and addressed. Also, fear of abandonment can bepart of a diagnosable personality disorder or other disorder that should be treated.

HEALING ABANDONMENT ISSUES

Once you recognize your fear of abandonment, there are some things you can do to begin healing.

Cut yourself some slack and stop the harsh self-judgment. Remind yourself of all the positive qualities that make you a good friend and partner.

Talk to the other person about your fear of abandonment and how it came to be. But be mindful of what you expect of others. Explain where you're coming from, but don't make your fear of abandonment something for them to fix. Don't expect more of them than is reasonable.

Work on maintaining friendships and building your support network. Strong friendships can boost yourself-worth and sense of belonging.

If you find this unmanageable, consider speaking to a qualified therapist. You may benefit from individual counseling.

How to Help Someone with Abandonment Issues

Here are a few strategies to try if someone you know is dealing with fear of abandonment:

- Start the conversation. Encourage them to talk about it, but don't presssure them.

- Whether it makes sense to you or not, understand that the fear is real for them.
- Assure them that you won't abandon them.
- Ask what you can do to help.
- Suggest therapy, but don't push it. If they express a desire to move forward, offer your assistance in finding a qualified therapist.

When to See a Doctor

If you've tried but can't manage your fear of abandonment on your own, or if you have symptoms of a panic disorder, anxiety disorder, or depression, see a healthcare provider.

You can start with your primary care physician for a complete checkup. They can then refer you to a mental health professional to diagnose and treat your condition.

Without treatment, personality disorders may lead to depression, substance use, and social isolation.

Effect on Relationships

The fear of abandonment is highly personalized. Some people are solely afraid of losing a romantic partner, others fear abandonment in other relationships.

To better explain how individuals with a fear of abandonment may navigate a relationship, here is an example of how a typical relationship may start and evolve. This example is especially true for romantic relationships, but there are many similarities in close friendships as well.

GETTING-TO-KNOW-ONE-ANOTHER

On getting to know one another, you feel relatively safe. You are not yet emotionally invested in the other person, so you continue to live your life while enjoying time with your chosen person.

Honeymoon Phase- This phase occurs when you make the choice to commit. You are willing to overlook possible red or yellow flags because you just get along so well. You start spending a great deal of time with the other person; and you always enjoy yourself. You start to feel secure.

Real Relationship - The honeymoon phase cannot last forever. No matter how well two people get along, real life always intervenes. People get sick, have family problems, start working difficult hours, worry about money, and need time to get things done.

Although this is a very normal and positive step in a relationship, it can be terrifying for those with a fear of abandonment who may see it as a sign that the other person is pulling away. If you have this fear, you are probably battling with yourself and trying very hard not to express your worries for fear of appearing clingy.

The Slight - People are human. They have moods and things on their minds. Regardless of how much they care for someone else, they cannot and should not be expected to always have that person at the forefront of their minds.

Especially once the honeymoon period is over, it is inevitable that a seeming slight will occur. This often takes the form of an unanswered text message, an unreturned phone call, or a request for a few days of alone time.

The Reaction -For those with a fear of abandonment, this is a turning point. If you have this fear, you are probably completely convinced that the slight is a sign that your partner no longer loves you. What happens next is almost entirely determined by the fear of abandonment, its severity, and the sufferer's preferred coping style.

Some people handle this by becoming clingy and demanding, insisting that their partner prove them love by jumping through hoops. Others run away, rejecting their partners before they are rejected. Still, others feel that the slight is their fault and attempt to transform themselves into the "perfect partner" in a quest to keep the other person from leaving.

In reality, the slight is most likely not a slight at all. Simply put, sometimes people just do things that their partners do not understand.

In a healthy relationship, the partner may recognize the situation for what it is—a normal reaction that has little or nothing to do with the relationship or they may feel upset by it, but address it with either a calm discussion or a brief argument. Either way, a single perceived slight does not become a dominating influence on the partner's feelings.

Partner's Point of View -From your partner's point of view, your sudden personality shift seems to come from out of left field. If your partner does not suffer from a fear of abandonment, they probably do not have the slightest idea as to why their previously confident, laid-back partner is suddenly acting clingy and demanding, smothering them with attention, or pulling away altogether.

Similar to phobias, it's impossible to simply talk or reason someone out of a fear of abandonment. No matter how many times your partner tries to reassure you, it will simply not be enough. Eventually, your behavior patterns and inconsolable reactions could drive your partner away, leading to the very conclusion that you fearmost.

ABOUT YOUR PARTNER WORKSHEET

The set of questions below is to be handled in a fun, conversational manner just to help you know more about your partner. It is specifically for bond building, nurturing growth, and showing commitment to understanding your partner better...have fun!

Fun and Games

What music did your partner listen to as a kid or teen?

What is your partner's ideal vacation spot?

Is there a TV show your partner is currently loving?

What upcoming events is your partner looking forward to?

Is there a book that has influenced your partner's life significantly?

The Future

How does your partner describe their ideal life?

Does your partner have a significant health or career goal?

What is your partner hoping to become better at in the next three years?

What are the most important items on your partner's bucket list?

Does your partner have an achievable long-term goal for their life?

You and Me

How did your partner discover they liked you?

What does your partner miss the most about you when you are apart?

What hopes does your partner have for your life in 3 years?

Can you describe a time your partner was proud of your relationship?

What activities or places does your partner love to do/visit with you?

Other People

Who is your partner's oldest friend?

Apart from you, who can your partner discuss their difficulties with?

Is there anyone who your partner sees as a role model?

Are they very close with any one relative? How do they catch up?

Does your partner see themselves as a sociable person?

Careers

What are your partner's friends like in the office?

What are they best at in their role?

What is their favorite thing about their role? Their least favorite thing?

How do they feel rewarded by their job, besides money?

How does their usual workday look, from start to finish?

Feelings

How does your partner unwind at the end of a long day?

What are the main feelings your partner has experienced today?

Is there anything in life that makes your partner really happy?

Does your partner consider themselves contented?

What are some things you do that make your partner feel great?

COPING STRATEGIES

If your fear is mild and well-controlled, you may be able to handle it simply by becoming educated about your tendencies and learning new behavior strategies. For most people, the fear of abandonment is rooted deeply in issues that are difficult to unravel with alone.

Professional assistance is often required to work through this fear and truly change your thoughts and behaviors.

Although treating the fear itself is critical, it is also essential to build a feeling of belonging. Rather than focusing all of your energy and devotion on a single partner, focus on building a community. No one-person can solve all of our problems or meet all of our needs. But a solid group of several close friends can each play an important role in ourlives.

Many people with a fear of abandonment state that they never felt like they had a "tribe" or a "pack" when they were growing up. For whatever reasons, they always felt "other" or disconnected from those around them but the good news is that it's never too late.

Whatever your current stage of life, it is important to surround yourself with other like-minded individuals. Make a list of your current hobbies, passions, and dreams. Then find others who share your interests.

While it istrue that not everyone who shares an interest will become a close friend, hobbies and dreams are an excellent stepping stone toward building a solid support network. Working on your passions also helps build self-confidence and the belief that you are strong enough to cope with whatever life throws your way.

JEALOUSY

There are times when jealousy affects the best among us. However, it is not always perceived the same. Different people may experience or display jealousy in contrasting fashion, owing largely to their personality types. But regardless, you need to understand that whether you believe being jealous is justified or not, it eventually ends up becoming a destructive influence, and will negatively affect your wellbeing.

What is jealousy? In it simplest form, jealousy can be defined as an emotion, or combination of emotions that manifest as either thought, actions or emotional feelings. It is believed that most people will experience feelings of jealousy at one-point or another in their lives, and while the reasons for jealousy are common among all walks of life, the expressions can vary significantly.

How to Identify if You Suffer from Jealousy

The appearance of jealousy may not always be obvious from an outside perspective, but traits are present that you would be able to identify. These include:

- **You Snoop:** This can include prying into private mail or email, screening phone calls, or just needing to know where your significant other or loved one is at all times. This can also include friends, who may be in contact with others you despise, causing you to feel left out.
- **Pettiness:** if you find yourself picking arguments for tiny things, and disguising it as "telling the truth", this is one of the signs of jealousy. On a subliminal level, the goal is to make the other person feel some of the emotions you are experiencing, but sugar coating it at the same time.
- **You Constantly Experience Doubts and Need Reassurance:** Eventually, a point is reached when your significant other/friend stops entertaining outbursts of jealousy, and this is when things take a new level. You may find yourself outright questioning that person if they still care about you, but are never convinced enough to listen to the reassurances. This could be a slippery slide down

to a very dark place, so try not to have your feelings of jealousy get this bad.

- **Insincerity:** Jealousy does not just stem from the belief that your partner is hiding an external relationship, but can also be triggered when the other person isuplifted. This can be as a result of a promotion, an extravagant gift from a relative, or anything that make the other person happy. You may say "congratulations" or "I'm happy for you", but your true feelings show through as insincerity.

Why Do Your Experience Jealousy?

Most of the causes of jealousy are common; meaning that if you experience it, the triggers are the same, regardless of cultural differences. These commonly include:

- **Insecurity:** Insecurity often does not just randomly appear [1], but develops slowly over a relationship. For example, if you notice your significant other publicly checking out other people, you develop some feelings of insecurity. Likewise, being uncomfortable with who you are, and then equating it with thefactthat you're not good enough for your partner can further in security.
- **Fear:** primarily the fear that your partner will leave you for someone better, may cause you to lash out and more publicly display jealousy. This could be the worst possible way to handle things, however, as lashing out due to fear will only serve to worsen things.
- **Competition:** completion in a relationshipis very common, even though you might like to believe that one person uplifts another. There is a constant battle on the low to see who is the "better" person in the relationship, which may lead to development of jealousy in at least one person. Not all competition is healthy competition, as we were taught in school.

Why Jealousy Is a Matter You Should be Concerned with

It is believed that a little jealousy is good, as it shows that youhave "interest" in your significant other, but this is not really the case. In fact, we all experience jealousy- that is a fact. But there are significant differences in the way we express our jealousy.

In fact, according to the Myers-Briggs Personalitytest (MBTI), differences in our personality type determine to a large extent the way we deal with jealousy. This is why some people seem unbothered by jealousy, or why some people do not see why their partner is acting out. On the other hand, some people experience a larger degree ofextroverted emotional feelings than others, whereby they wear their emotionsas a proud badge of honor.

At the end of it all, what you should beconcerned with is the way jealousy canalter your relationship. You can use it productively to change the way you handle your emotions, or let it run ok like wildfire and cause destruction, your choice.

How To Address Your Jealousy

- **Shift Your Point of View (POV):** sometime, staking a step back and trying to visualize if you're being fair can help you control your outbursts. It doesn't work for everyone, but is worth a shot.
- **Remind Yourself that you're Worth It:** if you feel undervalued, or underappreciated, you need to remind yourself that there are things you bring that no one else has to offer. Then, if you are 100% sure, you are not appreciated, leave a relationship where you are often belittled.
- **Practice Mindfulness:** Meditation can help you develop appreciation for the present, and boost self-control as well. This is a useful tool in minimizing jealous outbursts.
- **Seek Support When All Else Fails**: talk to a trusted friend, or a professional in an effort to get a foreign perspective. This can help you judge if your jealousy is unwarranted.

"Maybe he'll fall in love with his bubbly receptionist and leave me," "She's going to lunch with her ex-boyfriend, obviously she's still attracted to him," "He'll come home and tell me he wants a divorce," "Obviously she'll get the promotion! She is such a brown noser..." Whatever movie we have created in our heads, we will always find people or situations to support our story. What is the story you tell yourself? Do you believe that you are unlovable and soon your partner will find you out? What is at the core of your jealous feelings?

"Nothing can ruin a relationship faster than jealousy."

No one wants a jealous partner, sibling, colleague, or friend—and nobody enjoys feeling jealous or living out his or her jealousy with bizarre and hurtful behavior. Nothing can ruin a relationship faster than jealousy. The ever-pressing question is: How can we overcome it?

Solution 1: COMMUNICATION: Be emotionally intelligent with yourself first and those that are important to you, because no one can read your mind. If you are feeling jealous, be open with yourself about your intentions. Do you feel more deserving to be in that new position at work? Do you have cause to think your partner is cheating? Have you been cheatedonbefore? Very often we are unaware of what is going on subconsciously. It isuptoyouto find the root of your insecurity and then address it. Don't hide what it is—it doesn't have to be a deep secret that you carry.

Solution 2: TRUST: Jealousy comes out of a lack of trust; lack of trust in the process of life, in your partner, in yourself. Lack of trust breeds insecurity, which creates jealousy; we stifle these feelings because they are uncomfortable. It's a vicious circle, andas long as our thoughts and energy are clearly focused on what we could lose, that is exactly what will happen. This is the cold hard truth about jealousy: It's a self-fulfilling prophecy.

"It's a vicious circle, and as long as our thoughts and energy are clearly focused on what we could lose, that is exactly what will happen."

Solution 3: TAKE ACTION. It is paramount that we prevent ourselves from fixating on what we don't have and rather shift our perspective to the fact that our desires can and are revealing themselves through our daily actions. The big question and hard truth is, "How are we spending our days?" What we desire should be a source of inspiration, which provides us with the power, motivation, and ability to work toward and manifest (no matter how big or small).

If the green-eyed monster showshis face, remember that jealousy can be an extraordinarily powerful tool if we use it to propel ourselves to get what we most desire. Instead of being afflicted with envy, rather use this powerful energy of envy to help you work towards what will actually bring you more of what you desire and less of what you feel you lack.

"Emotions are simply something we experience, but we do not have to become them."

Emotions are simply something we experience, but we do not have to become them. See the jealousy you feel as a signal that something in you warrants your awareness, bring it to your consciousness and use it to bring about positive change; be it in your relationships with yourself or those you hold dearest to you.

The Danger of Jealousy

Jealousy doesn't become a problem until it's acted on. People that are prone to intense jealousy or possessiveness often harbor feelings of inadequacy or inferiority and have a tendency to compare themselves to others. Jealousy, at it score, is a by-product of fear, fear of not being good enough, fear of loss. When it hits, it can trick us into believing our relationship is in immediate danger, making it impossible to distinguish between natural feelings of protectiveness and irrational suspicion.

In other words, it's pretty terrible.

Yet the first time we see jealousy flare up in our partner, we may see it as "cute" and think, "Wow, this person must really love me!" If it's the healthy kind of jealousy, those feelings will fade without incident and without negatively impacting the relationship. But we must be on alert for early warning signs of unhealthy behavior because it can lead to other forms of abuse.

Unhealthy relationships often start with small things like a suspicious partner hunting for evidence of cheating. If they show up empty, rather than feel satisfied, they'll vent their frustration through a variety of methods while breaking down their S.O.'s self-esteem with accusations, blaming, name-calling, and threats before moving on to emotional and physical abuse. Their tactics take on many forms, but as their jealousy grows, so does the chance for escalation. That's why it's important to identify red flags early.

What Unhealthy Jealousy Looks Like

It is vey easy to confuse unhealthy jealous behavior with love. Below are common warning signs that often show up at the start of relationships and snowball into dangerous problems later on.

You're Expected to Spend All YourTime with Them

They're not just excited to see you, they're insistent. They ask you to blow off practice, ditch your friends, or back out of work, school, or family commitments because they've "never felt this way before" and "need to be near you." They may become pouty/whiny when you don't comply, and they tend to show up wherever you are, uninvited. They hate being away from you and contact you constantly when you're not together.

While it may seem sweet when someone wants to spend all of their time with you, a person who respects you will understand that you need time away from the relationship and you deserve time to be alone and pursue other interests- without facing punishment for it.

A caring partner will never force you to give up your hobbies, relationships, jobs, or activities so they can dominate your time.

You're Required to Check-In

Your significant other likes to know where you are. They like to know what you're doing and who you're with. When you're away, they call, text, or contact you throug social media expecting immediate responses. They ask you to turn on tracking apps, like Snap Maps, and so they can see where you are. You keep your phone close at hand because you know if you don't reply fast enough, they'll become suspicious or get upset.

When we care about someone, its normal to ask for a text or phone call in situations where we want to know they're safe. For example, we may ask them to text us when they make it home- that's normal. An S.O. expecting you to keep him/her a breast of your every move anytime you're apart is not.

A healthy relationship doesn't require "check-in's." Your partner shouldn't require you to stay in constant contact when you're away, and no one should ever insist on tracking you with anapp or any other means. Knowing you're safe should be enough, and if it's not, your boundaries are not being respected. You are your own person, and you're allowed to live your own life.

There Are Rules about Who You Can Talk to

You know there are certain peopleyou'renot allowed to interact with unless you want to fight with your partner; the list might include exes, people you used to have a crush on, that flirty co-worker, etc. The reasons you're not allowed to talk to each person varies: "I trust you, I just don't trust them," "It makes me uncomfortable when you talk to that ex," "I just think I should be enough for you," "I've seen the way he/she looks at you." The list goes on, andyou go along with it even though you don't agree because it's not worth the fight.

Demands about who you can talk to can lead to an abuse tactic called isolation. What begins with not being able to talk to a certain person becomes rules about staying away from pretty much anyone they feel is in competition for your affection, time, or attention. Eventually, everyone becomes off-limits until you are isolated to only your partner, paving the way for depression and possibly an environment for physical abuse.

It's never okay to regulate who your partner can and can't talk to. Part of loving someone means trusting them to make good decisions about the company they keep. You can vocalize your concerns in a loving, honest way, but then you must trust your partner's judgment. If one of you can't trust the other, it may be time to move on.

They're Suspicious

If you go out with friends, you know you're going to get the third degree from your partner after. Your S.O. worries when you're away and is convinced everyone is flirting with you. Sometimes it only takes someone else looking at you for them to get upset, and then they act as though you're to blame. You get accused of being too friendly, dressing too provocatively, or giving people "the wrong idea." No matter how much you reassure them of your faithfulness, they never believe you.

People in healthy relationships don't put their partner's every move under the microscope. They don't constantly doubt the other's intentions or laden them with accusatory questions. Love doesn't scour for evidence or assume wrongdoing–insecurity does.

If you or your S.O. struggles with on-going suspicion, there may be a deeper underlying issue, and the relationship won't work until it's dealt with. Love withers whenever suspicion out weighs trust.

They're Possessive

They've given you jewelry or a personal memento they want you to wear all the time so people know you're taken. Even if they're not overly touchy in private, they're big on public displays of affection, particularly if your exes around. They're all over your social media and insist on having profile pictures and status updates together. They're hostile to someone they think wants to date you. They've made you leave parties or cancel plans to be with them and make statements like, "You're mine," or "No one will ever love you like I do."

Movies and books have a bad habit of romanticizing this behavior; in real life, a possessive partner's goal is not to share you with anyone. They operate from a need for control and will try to manipulate you emotionally, using gifts, over-the-top gestures, and compliments to re-establish your "belonging" to them. Their obsession can lead to physical confrontations with people they view as competition, and as their behavior continues, they won't shy away from humiliating you in public if it means asserting their dominance; for example, they may yell at you and grab your arm to make you leave a gathering. With possessiveness, physical abuse and isolation aren't far behind.

People in happy, committed relationships understand love requires letting their significant other have space to be their own person. They let go of the need to mark their territory or to scare off the competition because they trust each other.

They Have a QuickTemper

One minute you're looking forward to dinner at your favorite restaurant, next your partner's causing a scene because you arrived a few minutes late. This happens pretty often, but you blame yourself because you know your partner has buttons that send them into a rage, and it's your fault for pressing them. You wish you could be a better girlfriend/boyfriend, but you keep messing up, giving them a reason to explode. Some days you feel lucky they're so forgiving and still love you at all because you make so many mistakes, even when you're being careful.

If your partner's temper is quick on the draw, it's not a reflection of you. It simply means they haven't learned how to deal with conflict or they may be using it as a means to manipulate, control, or dominate you. Either way, it's not your fault.

Healthy relationships work hard at conflict resolution. They're dedicated to finding ways to talk through problems without hurting or disrespecting the other person. If the reaction you're met with is always anger, it's not your responsibility to stay and be an emotional, verbal, or physical outlet for it, that's not love.

They Monitor Your Communications

Your partner tells you they're an open book and want absolutely no secrets between the two of you. That'swhy they require the passwords to your phone, email account, Facebook, SnapChat, Instagram, and any social media app you use. They go through your messages, question you about conversations, mince sover your words, and delete contacts they don't approve of, with or without your consent. Sometimes you notice your password doesn't work or you've been lockedout of your own account. You tell yourself it's no big deal; it's a small price to pay tobe with them and show them they can trust you.

Wanting your passwords is not about love, it's about dominance and control. Yourpasswordsare yours alone, and anyone insisting you supply this information doesn't trust you and is acting in a controlling manner.

Healthy relationships don't require you to prove your trustworthiness because trust doesn't require proof. Even if you don't mind sharing the information, indulging this negative behavior is communicating that it's okay to violate your privacy, opening the door to other abusive behaviors down the road.

They're Emotionally Intense

You noticed your partner came on strong right from the beginning, but you figured it was because they liked you so much so now, they hate being apart. They call and text you constantly and comb through all your social media accounts, liking and/or commenting on everything, even posts that are years old. They always want to have you to themselves and were quick to say "I love you," though it felt fast. Conversations about "forever" come up a lot, and they talk about how they would "go crazy," "die," or "kill" themselves if the two of you ever broke up. It can be hard to get away from them, andyou sometimes think they're following you.

While it can be flattering to think someone adores us so intensely, beneath the surface is emotional dependency. If they come on too strong from the beginning, that same neediness may turn into pushy physical advances, stalking, threats of self-harm, and/or violence.

Happy couples know they cannot be everything to their partner. Each person needs a certain level of freedom and independence, which is why you should never beheld accountable for another person's happiness. Emotional intensity often elicits a feeling of suffocation, and if you are feeling this way, don't ignore it.

HOW TO STOP JEALOUSY

The key to maintaining a healthy relationship isto spot the signs early. If your partner displays jealous tendencies, here are some first steps you can take to try to navigate the situation:

Talk to your partner about their concerns, taking a gentle approach. Listen to what they have to say and be honest about how their actions are making you feel.

Establish boundaries with your partner. Communicate how you want to be treated, taking into consideration what's important to each of you. For example, let them know you can contact them once when you arrive at a friend's house, but that you will not be checking your phonethe entire night. Knowing what the expectations are will alleviate guess work and anxiety for both of you.

Once you've talked through it, it's time to show your partner a little extra love. They may be feeling vulnerable, so don't hold back on the affection. Let them know you appreciate their honesty and any concessions they've made.

As you will likely have to revisit the conversation several times before both parties are fully comfortable, continue to be patient but also firm about your boundaries. If you can't come to a compromise, it may be time to end things.

Unhealthy Relationship Behavior: Jealousy

Jealousy is a feeling, not a call to action. When it creeps up, take a deep breath and remind yourself that a feeling is

Not the same as reality. In otherwords, just because you worry someone is cheating doesn't mean they are.

When you focus on something, it expands, so if you've convinced yourself that your partner is cheating, you'll see evidence where there is none. Instead of obsessing, acknowledge the feeling, then let it be. If we don't give it extra attention, it will usually pass on its own.

Ask yourself what you stand to gain from jealous inclinations. Will acting on your impulses hurt or improve the relationship? Will it make you feel better or worse? Will it fix the problem or aggravate it?

Accept that in relationships, there is no certainty. Just as you cannot make someone love you, you cannot make someone remain loyal or stay. If you're unable to trust your partner, you're better off moving on so you can enjoy independence or find someone else who shares your values.

If you can't move past a jealous feeling, be honest. Instead of pouting or giving the silent treatment, tell your partner specifically what is making you feel that way and listen to their response. You'll likely find the interaction strengthens the relationship rather than tears it down the way punishments and games do.

When you Friend Needs Help

If your friend is in a relationship and you see the warning signs, keep this in mind:

- Don't be afraid to speak up. Often, it's not as obvious to the person it's happening to, so approach them in a caring manner.
- Don't be forceful or get angry if they disagree with your assessment; it may take time for them to see things from an objective perspective.
- Make yourself available so that when they're ready to talk, they'll know you're there for them.
- Continue to love them through their difficult situation and vocalize about yourconcerns.

If you suspect your friend is in a dangerous situation, contact another trusted friend or adult, and refer to the National Domestic Abuse Hotline for tips athttp://www.thehotline.org

WRAPPING UP

Real love is not possessive. It does not act out of dominance, fear, or control. Rather, it is a mutual admiration and respect for another human being we long to see happy and whole. In a healthy relationship, there is a balance between compromise, self-love, and consideration for the other person.

While jealousy is a natural feeling everyonegetsfrom time to time, whenwe obsess over it, it can change us and end relationships. It's important to recognize when jealousy is motivating unhealthy behaviors and to protect our boundaries before they get crossed. Speaking up early will decrease the chance of escalation and will help lasting love blossom in healthy soil where trust runs deep, respect is present, and communication is abundant.

If your partner's jealousy takes a turn toward abuse, talk to someone right away! Tell a friend, family member, or a trusted adult. Ending an abusive relationship can be a dangerous and scary time, so be sure to gather the support you need and visit http://www.thehotline.org for additional guidance on how to remain safe.

PART TWO: JUMP-OFF YOUR HEALING AND DEEPEN YOUR RELATIONSHIP

CHAPTER 4: TIME TO STOP STEALING THE MAGIC

First, let's talk about how your brain gets wired to create anxiety in the firstplace. Well, some people are born with the propensity for an anxious brain. So that means there's a familial preisposition, brains do not fall far from the tree. If your parents have anxiety, then you may also have anxiety too. Therefore, our brains are wired like our parent's brains but secondly is the environment; nature and nurture. The nurture part is if you feel anxious and you use the anxiety brain pattern. You are hard wiring that pattern into your brain every time you use it. Continue reading to learn how to re-wire your brain.

What Does this Anxiety Brain Map Look Like?

There are five main speeds in our brain to be able to shift in and out of states that we need to and we want to get in each day. The first speed is the extra slow speed that's what keeps you asleep. Slow speed is the one that shifts you into sleep. Medium speed is couch mode and that's the speed you use when you're relaxing on the sofa. Fast speed is the perfect speed for information. So that's the speed that your brain uses when you go to school or work. The fifth speed is the fastest speed and it's used when something stressful happens in yourlife.

Today the main struggle for most people is going into fight or flight mode and gets stuck in this mode. So you must be able to get out of that mode to feel focused and relaxed.

TECHNIQUE 1: CHANGING YOURSELF TO REDUCE TOXICITY IN YOUR RELATIONSHIP

First of all, there is a very complex and scientific law, which is called Hebb's Law. This law shows that neurons that fire together wire together. So every time you use that brain pattern, it is hardwiring itself in. Basically, when you continue to use the same brain pattern it's creating neural pathways in your brain. Therefore, neuropath ways are similar to roads, streets, or paths. Every time you use the anxiety brain pattern you're trampling over the weeds and creating this divot that is memorizing the pattern.

The key to success is to take Hebb's Law and use it to create a new path of calm and focus. So how do we do that, there's a method called amphibian homeostatic learning. This works by stopping the use of the harmful brain pattern that creates your anxiety. Therefore, basically unwiring that brain pattern to create a healthy new one. So we're unwiring, rewiring and that's happening simultaneously to get rid of anxiety.

What do You have to do to Rewire Your Brain?

It's simple but maybe not easy. The simplicity lies in how we can approach getting rid of anxiety by rewiring your brain in two ways.

Number one, a top-down approach that's neuro feedback brain training. Neuro feedback can unwire that anxious brain pattern and rewire that calm and focus brain pattern without you doing anything. It teaches your brain to make calmer focus speed and to make less of that extra fast speed. Therefore, it literally shifts your brain out of that anxiety mode and creates more clam focus for you.

Number two is you have to use your mind and your body for a bottom-up approach to rewiring your brain. We know that anxiety many times can be partially in nature and a lot more nurture. Meaning that the constant use of the anxiety pattern is really what's wiring it. So using behavioral techniques to use your mind and your body to calm yourself down. However, meaning that you have to change your behaviors, you have to force yourself to be able to do the thing that you may struggle with. This step becomes so much easier when using neuro feedback because your brain is moving into a calmer mode. Then that enables you to be able to use some of these behavioral techniques.

The rewiring of your brain is a result of neuroplasticity, which includes two things: Neurogenesis (thegrowth of new neurons) and synaptogeneis (new connections between neurons). You can enhance the growth of those two things through meditation, reflectivese lf-inquiry, mindfulness and asking meaningful questions and visualization.

Through visualization, you can turn an abstract hope into a picture that not only inspires you, but also guides you. According to a study called "The Future of Memory: Remembering, Imagining and the Brain," by Daniel L Schacter, Donna Rose Addis, and Karl K. Szpunar.The human brain can't always distinguish between a memory and a vision of the future.

In other words, when you envision your end goal, you and your brain can work towards recreating it in real life.

VISUALIZATION

Your brain believes what you imagine. Brain science reveals that you experience real-world and imaginary actions in similar ways. For example, whether you are acing an event or only picturing it, you activate many of the same neural networks and pathways of nerve cells that link your body to the brain impulses that control it. What's on your mind screen stimulates the sympathetic nervous system, which activates an increase in heart rate, breathing, and blood pressure. Just by envisioning a movement, such as holding hands with your partner-to-be, elicits nervous-system responses of that same action.

Go ahead and imagine yourself holding the hand of your beloved – as if it's happening right now. Then, get even more detailed in your visualization. As if you are watching a scene or interaction of your beloved in your own movie – where you are the star. Let all your senses come alive. What are you feeling, hearing, smelling, tasting and touching in this beautiful scene? Are you walking hand-in-hand on a gorgeous beach while on vacation together? Are you in a kitchen making dinner and laughing hysterically? Maybe it's a quiet scene where both of you are cuddled up on the couch reading books?

Allow yourself to really surrender into this visualization, sensing it and feeling it all. It feels good, right? To make this extra powerful, visualize this everyday for at least 2 minutes. Add in more details each time and increase your imagination play to 5 minutes per day. Smile and bask in the feelings of joy and peace, and of feeling so deeply loved and adored by your partner.

The more you envision, the more you activate your emotions to match the scene on your mind screen. The more detailed you get in your visualization with your beloved, the more familiar you become to achieving it because you are creating new neuro pathways in your brain. Plus, your nervous system reaps the benefits: increase in calm and confidence and decrease in heart rate and stress hormones. So, what are you waiting for? Give visualization a try!

Step One: Imagine your perfect lazy Sunday with your ideal partner.

To really get into this one, take a moment to sit down comfortably with your back supported and your head free.

Take a few slow, deep breaths, then close your eyes. Now, imagine waking up and rolling over and seeing your ideal partner lying next to you, fast asleep.

Take a moment and really picture what they look like: What color is their hair? What do they look like when they're sleeping? Can you hear their breathing? Let your imagination run wild.

Now, they wake up and open their eyes and they see you and make eye contact. Notice what color their eyes are, and notice what their smile looks like when they seeyou.

They pull the covers away and you see their body as they walk to the bathroom. How tall are they? What physical form do they take? Just see them as they walk through the room.

As you both wake up and start the day, imagine what your activities look like. Do you go out for brunch or do you cook at home? If you cook at home, who cooks and what do you make?

Smell the food in the air and see it on the table in front of you. Picture the table itself. Do you sit in front of the TV or in front of each other? Is your table in your kitchen or on your balcony?

As you're chatting over brunch, notice what the conversation is about and what attributes about your partner come out when they talk? Do they like to talk about politics or work? What kind of job do they have? Do they want kids?

You wrap up brunch and head out for your perfect Sunday. Just imagine what that is for you both: Hiking, exploring the city, going to see a movie, going for a long drive?

Throughout the day, notice the moments that you connect and that you make eye contact. Notice what it feels like when you're riding in the car and you reach over and touch their hand. Is their skin soft or rough; do they hold your hand back?

Now, imagine that the day is winding down and you're back home getting ready for bed. I want you to have some fun here and picture your ideal sexual encounter with this person.

Are you in the bed or on the dining room table? Are you wearing anything? Are there rose petals or candles? Really take the time to see the images, smell the smells, taste the tastes, and feel the feelings.

Then imagine yourself falling asleep in their arms, feeling safe and connected and so incredibly grateful for the bond that you have with this person.

Taking a nice, deep inhale, savoring all of those feelings and images. As you exhale, bring yourself back to the present.

How did that feel? Was it dreamy and perfect, or did you have difficulty picturing many of the details? If it's the latter, that's OK. Because I'm about to give you a piece of homework to help you really hone in on the details of your ideal partner.

Step Two: Writedown 100 attributes you would want your ideal partner to have.

The items on the list should be more than "nice" or "kind." Be sure to write out the full 100. Even if you get to 60 and think that you're done, keep going! If you feel stuck, think back to the visualization.

The reason it's important to be specific is because the universe can't deliver your desires if you don't ask for them. If you go to a restaurant and order "food," the waiter will be confused and won't know what to bring you. The same goes for your love life.

Step Three: Throw out your list.

The next part of this exercise is to take the list you just wrote and throw it out. Yep! Burn it, toss it into the closet, tear it up into little pieces.

You're doing this because the purpose of this assignment isn't to try to control every little detail; it's just to get to the core of what you want.

You place the order, and then you trust that the chef will bring you something that's in line with what you specified, even if you don't know exactly what the food will look like or what kind of plate it will come on or how many minutes it will take to arrive. Let go of your attachment to the outcome.

Step Four: Last but not least, make sure you're fulfilled.

There's one other key aspect of this process, and that's making sure that you are 100 percent fulfilled before you try to bring someone else into your life.

Many of us subscribe to the 80/20 rule. We believe that if we're 80 percent fulfilled, our partner can bring the other 20. But it doesn't work that way because happiness is an inside job.

So your home work is to find tools and techniques to get you to the place where you feel 100 percent fulfilled on your own. I want you to spend the next seven days leaving your house like the 100 percent fulfilled version of you. Do your hair, buy some new clothes that make you feel great, take baths, participate in your favorite hobbies, etc. Because when you feel your best, other people are automatically drawn to you.

I know this might seem like a lot, but I assure you that doing the groundwork now will help you in the long run as you navigate the beautiful, messy world of love. Take the time to get really specific about your desires, and then throw the rest to the universe.

How to Practice Visualization

1. **Know what you want** - To manifest the kind of life you wish for, it would be great to have a clear idea of your wants and why. You can achieve this by wt you value and what makes you happy most in your life. Ever had that moment when you feel joy and happy while doing a certain thing? If yes, then that is a great sign of something you should want in your life.

   Ask yourself: if there is nothing holding me back, what would I love to see in my life?

2. **Describe your vision in details** - When you want to personify the life you want you should have a clear picture of how it should look like. You can jot it down for memory sake. It would help you know the kind of life you want, making it more precise and easy for you to achieve.

3. **Start visualizing and create the emotions** - When you are ready, you can start imagining the result. Start to imagine the pleasure, the

rhythms, the sensational smell, and even the taste of achieving your desire. Don't forget to feel those emotions that accompany it. Feel it as if the life you are imagining is real.

Ask yourself: how would I feel, if all my imaginations and come to pass?

4. **Take daily actions** - The life you wish to bring to pass won't be created in a day, just like the saying "Rome wasn't built in a day," but with series of hard work towards your goal. Don't be lost in how far you've gone, instead focus on the present and make sure you meet your daily or weekly goals to reach the life you want.

Ask yourself: what is that thing I can do today that would get me closer to the life I want?

5. **Have grit and persevere** - When creating the life you want, you'll be faced with series of challenges. In fact, one thing you should do when visualizing is also to imagine all the unforeseen challenges and how to overcome them, which is the most important thing to do.

Ask yourself: what should I do that would help me persevere when I am facing those challenges?

In order to rewire your brain for the long term, you must practice visualization for at least six weeks for just five to 10 minutes a day.

If you're busy during the day, try doing the practice before going to bed or first thing in the morning. Before you start the visualization process, ask yourself the questions below:

- What is my unique talent?
- Who would benefit?
- What is my passion?
- What is my higher calling?
- What are my goals?

It's important to imagine who you want to be or what you want to accomplish. For example, you might want to deliver an amazing presentation that will impress your boss. Think about yourself walking up to the front of the office and speaking with confidence, and then receiving a standing ovation.

Now that you have this image in mind, you simply must match your "memory" or "vision" of it happening. If you want to get a stellar year-end review from your manager, write down that goal on a sticky note and then read it every morning. You'll then move throughout your day with this intention in mind.

Experts have yet to determine the limits of the brain's abilities. Some believe that we may never fully understand them all. But evidence does support the existence of one of its most important processes: neuroplasticity.

"Neuroplasticity" refers to your brain's ability to restructure or rewire itself when it recognizes the need for adaption. In other words, it would continue developing and changing throughout life.

For example, if brain trauma after a car accident affects your ability to speak, you haven't necessarily lost this ability permanently. Therapy and rehabilitation could help your brain relearn this ability by repairing old path ways or creating new ones.

WHAT IS THE MEANING OF NEUROPLASTICITY?

It refers to the physiological changes in the brain that happen as the result of our interactions with our environment. From the time the brain begins to develop in the uteros until the day we die, the connections among the cells in our brains reorganize in response to our changing needs. This dynamic process allows us to learn from and adapt to different experiences

Our brains are truly extraordinary; unlike computers, which are built to certain specifications and receive software updates periodically, our brains can actually receive hardware updates in addition to software updates. Different pathways form and fall dormant, are created and are discarded, according to our experiences.

When we learn something new, we create new connections between our neurons. We rewire our brains to adapt to new circumstances. This happens on a daily basis, but it's also something that we can encourage and stimulate.

THE THEORY AND PRINCIPLES OF NEUROPLASTICITY

Before we get too ahead of ourselves, let's take a moment to look at the theory and principles underpinning neuroplasticity.

First, we should note that, although we have a fairly succinct definition of neuroplasticity above, the reality is a bit less well-defined. Neuroplasticity experts Christopher A. Shaw and Jill C. McEachern describe it thisway:

"While many neuroscientists use the word neuroplasticity as an umbrella term, it means different things to researchers in different subfields... In brief, a mutually agreed upon framework does not appear to exist"

Neuroplasticity is one fundamental process that describes any change in final neural activity or behavioral response, or;

Neuroplasticity is an umbrella term for a vast collection of different brain changes and adaptation phenomena.

The first perspective lends itself to a single theory of neuroplasticity with some basic principles, and that research on the subject would contribute to a single, all-inclusive framework of neuroplasticity. The second perspective would require numerous different frameworks and systems to understand each phenomenon.

Unfortunately, there is still no unifying theory of neuroplasticity that I can lay out in simple terms here. All I can say with certainty is that this is still a young field and new finding are popping up everyday.

What we do know right now is that there are two main types of neuroplasticity:

Structural neuroplasticity, in which the strength of the connections between neurons (or synapses) changes.

Neuroplasticity and Psychology

These new lines of research are exciting for neuroscientists, biologists, and chemists, but they are also exciting for psychologists.

In addition to changes in the way the brain works and functional adaptations, neuroplasticity offers potential avenues for psychological change as well.

WHAT IS COGNITIVE BEHAVIOUR THERAPY?

Cognitive behaviour therapy (CBT) is an effective treatment approach for a range of mental and emotional health issues, including anxiety and depression. CBT aims to help you identify and challenge unhelpful thoughts and to learn practical self-help strategies. These strategies are designed to bring about immediate positive changes in your quality of life.

CBT can be good for anyone who needs support to challenge unhelpful thoughts that are preventing them from reaching their goals or living the life they want to live.

CBT aims to show you how your thinking affects your mood. It teaches you to think in a less negative way about yourself and your life. It is based on the understanding that thinking negatively is a habit that, like any other habit, can be broken.

When CBT is Useful

CBT is used to treat a range of psychological problems including:

- Anxiety
- Anxiety disorders such as social phobia, obsessive-compulsive disorder or post-traumatic stress disorder
- Depression
- Low self-esteem
- Irrational fears
- Hypochondria
- Substance misuse, such as smoking, drinking or other drug use
- Problem gambling
- Eating disorders
- Insomnia
- Marriage or relationship problems

Certain emotional or behavioural problems in children or teenagers.

Using CBT to Treat Anxiety

Everyone feels anxious sometimes. Anxiety serves as a means of protection and can increase your performance in stressful situations. For example, the rush of anxiety that often occurs before a job interview or a big race can enhance your performance.

But for some people, the feeling of anxiety is more general. This means that you always feel on alert or fearful no matter what activity you are doing. This can be extremely distressing and get in the way of your daily life.

If your level of anxiety begins to interfere with your ability to function, it is important that you begin to learn some skills for coping with these anxious feelings. This is where CBT can help. It focuses on changing patterns of thinking and beliefs that are associated with, and trigger, anxiety.

Using CBT to Treat Depression

People with depression can have ongoing negative feelings about themselves, other people and the world around them. This negative thinking pattern can become automatic so that they don't notice when their judgement is irrational or unfair on themselves.

CBT can help people with depression by giving them tools to challenge the negative thoughts and override them with more realistic and positive thought processes.

CBT is also used to help many more psychological problems. In some cases, other forms of therapy used at the same time are recommended for best results. Talk to your doctor for further information and advice.

CBT and Thoughts, Feelings and Behaviours

The main focus of CBT is that thoughts, feelings and behaviours combine to influence a person's quality of life. For example, severe shyness in social situations (social phobia) may come from the person thinking that other people will always find them boring or stupid. This belief could cause the person to feel extremely anxious in social situations.

This could lead to a specific behavior in social situations, such as trembling, sweating, accelerated heartrate or other uncomfortable symptoms. The person could then feel overwhelmed with negative emotions (such as shame) and negative self-talk ('I'm such anidiot'). Their fear of social situations could become worse with every bad experience.

CBT aims to teach people that it is possible to have control over their thoughts, feelings and behaviours. CBT helpsthe person to challenge and overcome automatic beliefs, and use practical strategies to change or modify their behaviour. The result is more positive feelings, which in turn lead to more positive thoughts and behaviours.

CBT focuses on changing unhelpful or unhealthy thoughts and behaviours. It is a combination of two therapies: 'cognitive therapy' and 'behaviour therapy'. The basis of both these techniques is that healthy thoughts lead to healthy feelings and behaviours.

YOUR HIGHER SELF

Seeing yourself in higher light is the key to creating the desired changes in your life. Learning to see yourself in higher light is required to create yourself a new. Without the ability to envision yourself doing something you currently can't, you will never do it. The vision of yourself doing something you want will be the focal point of your motivation as you move forward. Without the vision, the motivation is lost; without the motivation, the desire will remain unfulfilled. The unity of vision and desire leads to success.

The key to self-improvement is seeing oneself in higher light. The components of seeing yourself in higher light are: maintaining a positive lense towards yourself, believing in yourself, letting go of negative beliefs, and believing you are without fault. Maintaining a positive lens towards yourself will allow youto maintain vision. Believing in yourself is key to keeping your focus. Letting go of negative beliefs ensures you do not stop yourself from seeing yourself positively. Believing you are without fault is part of seeing yourself in higher light.

Seeing yourself in higher light requires maintaining a positive lens. Looking at yourself and seeing the best parts of yourself is the way to be who you want to be. Placing your attention on your positive aspects is how these aspects will grow. Focusing on the parts of yourself you love is the way to see yourself in higher light. Motivating yourself completely requires you to look at yourself with the feeling of love. Being very clear as to why you are doing something is critical to maintaining motivation through the struggle.

The next step is believing in yourself. Self-belief is critical to going your own way, maintaining focus, and going the distance to achieve your goals. Self-belief enables you to walk the path with confidence you are headed in the right direction. Believing in yourself will allow you to do what is required. Self-belief gives you the fortitude to go great length in achieving your goals.

Letting go of your negative beliefs is the most important step in seeing yourself in higher light. Your negative beliefs cloud your vision, undermine yourself-belief, and stop you from being your best self. Letting go of them will stop all of this. This can be accomplished through an easy to perform meditation. The meditation involves working with your HigherSelf to bring to light your most harmful negative beliefs. Your Higher Self can then release these beliefs and help you amplify new positive beliefs as well.

The way to see yourself in the highest light possible is to believe you are without fault. There is nothing wrong with the way you are being. The way you are being is perfect in every way. When you adopt this view of yourself, you create the means to allow yourself to become this way in the future. Seeing yourself in this light is the way to let go of your faults. The faults you have, serve a purpose. Their purpose is to allow you to discover you are faultless. Once you no longer see your current state as containing faults, the faults beg into disappear. Being without shame helps you to see yourself as faultless. Without the shame attached, the corresponding state of being is able to be released. The way to see yourself in higher light is to be free of shame.

8 WAYS TO DEVELOP A MORE POSITIVE ATTITUDE

What if there was a way you could easily expand your mind and see greater possibilities in life? What if you could develop better skills naturally?

When people think of having a positive attitude, they probably think it's little more than plastering a smile on their face and trying to think happy thoughts.

But it's more than that.

A positive attitude is something that goes deeper and has an effect beyond surface cheer. Negative attitudes promote fear, and a narrowing of focus and the mind, while positive attitudes do the opposite. No one should live in a constant state of "fight or flight", but negative attitudes create exactly that scenario.

Studies have also shown that having a true positive attitude makes your view of life seem broad, full of possibilities. That view leads to actually living your life in a way that makes it natural to be exposed to and acquire new skills.

Here are some ways to maintain a positive attitude in the workplace, regardless of whether it comes naturally or not:

1. Surround Yourself with Positive People

The old saying "birds of a feather flock together" can be viewed in two ways. Either people who are similar naturally find each other, or people in a group become the same overtime.

Who you hang around with rubs off on you. If you're always with negative people who complain about everything, you'll become a complainer and see the world as negative as they do. You might think you can stay positive and change them, but that's not going to be the case. Try to connect with people who like their job, have new ideas, and are interested in lots of other things besides work. It'll make your whole outlook better.

You can't always pick your co-workers, but you can be cautious about how much time you spend with them, and in what setting. If you're stuck with a negative bunch, be careful not to participate in the negativity. Take breaks and go for a walk rather than immerse yourself in negative breakroom drama and gossip.

2. Fill your Mind with Positive Input

The same way that the people you are around change you to be more like them, so is what you feed your mind.

Listen to positive music with headphones. Listen to uplifting audio books on the drive into work. Read books that are encouraging. Watch videos and listen to podcasts that are positive or help you improve skills.

If you are what you eat holds true for your body, your mind is what you feed it.

3. Control your Language

No, this isn't about the language police, or trying to swear less (although the latter is probably a good idea). This is about being conscious of the words you use when speaking and thinking.

The Sapir-Whorf hypothesis (which played heavily into the recent movie "Arrival") suggests that the structure of language affects a person's view of the world, and the way they think. Taken to the furthest extent, your language actually limits ordelineates how you are able to perceive the world.

It's an hypothesis, granted. But on a smaller level, the language you use everyday, both in thought and spoken word, has a cumulative effect on how you think about yourself, your work, and those aroundyou.

This may seem like a silly example, but it might be the difference between seeing your day as filled with tasks, or filled with opportunities. The former is tiring and arduous, making you feel trapped in a daily grind. The latter is exciting with potential.

Be aware of how you choose to think and speak at work. Find a positive way to view everything and everyone.

4. Create a Routine for the Day

Routines get a bad rap. It's easy to think that if you have a routine at work, you're stuck in a rut or you're not "flexible". The truth is, though, that routines give us good fall-back structure. A morning routine is especially good, since for many people, the morning is both when we're most alert and awake yet sometimes notable to buckle down and get started.

Create a routine that helps you get the most important work done, take breaks at the right time, and leaves the last hour or so of the work day for less arduous work and preparation for the next day. Most of us get tired by the end of the day, so don't leave tough work for then. It's important to end each day by getting prepared for the next.

5. Be Nice to Other People

Being kind to other people makes you happy. A study in the Journal of Social Psychology found that doing something kind for people has the same effect as trying new and exciting things when it comes to feeling happy.

Even better?

A study in the Journal of Happiness Studies found that the memory of doing something kind for someone causes us to want to do it again.

If you make being nice to other people a regular thing, it'll become a cycle of generosity and happiness that makes you feel good and causes those around you to feel happy as well.

Think of the worst negative work environment possible. Negativity feeds on more negativity until it seems overwhelming. Be nice to other people and watch them pay it forward.

If your work is difficult and you can't get away from that, and finding a positive attitude about the work itselfis a challenge, be kind to thepeople around you and let that be an effective substitute.

Appreciating and recognizing co-workers can go a long way in making your day better.

6. Don't Rely on an Outside Source of Positivity

Carry a positive attitude with you. Think of a positive attitude like a survival tool: carry it with you at all times for emergencies.

Whether you rely on a phrase that you repeat over and over when times are stressful or you have some other trick to help resurrect and keep a positive attitude, be sure to come up with a mechanism that doesn't rely on someone else or a specific situation.

7. Create High Points in Each Day and Week

One of the best parts of an exciting vacation is the days leading up to it, when you have it to look forward to. Knowing something good is coming can make otherwise dreary days more bearable.

You can create the same effect by creating small "high points" in each day to help you get through projects or days that might otherwise seem draining. This is why taking breaks is important, but not every break is as valuableas they couldbe.

A few suggestions:

- Don't turn to unhealthy food as a reward. You'll end up with negative effects and a bad habit for junk food or excessive coffee.
- Take breaks outside or away from work when possible.
- Consider a walk, solitude, silence — whatever sounds good and is doable where you work.
- Find a place to read a book not related to work.

Daily high points should be small and simple, not requiring money or creating a habit that could have negative effects on your health or budget if you do them every day (e.g. walk to the bakery for a donut and coffee every day). Weekly or monthly high points can be a bit bigger. Maybe every Thursday you eat lunch at a restaurant nearby instead of bringing in yourown lunch. Whatever it is, create something to look forward to.

8. Assume Responsibility, and Choose your Response

Refusing to take responsibility for your actions and your situation, or not taking control of how you respond, kills a positive attitude immediately.

Afterall, if something happens and you're at fault or in some way responsible, refusing to acknowledge it means you can't correct the behavior and it will happen again, andyou also set yourself up for a victimhood mindset in which things happen toyou.

You will be more positive seeing life as something you have some control over rather than at the mercy of fate. Think of it as an equation: $E + R = O$ (event + response = outcome). How you respond has an effect on the outcome, even when events are out of your control.

The pursue-withdraw pattern is destructive and if not addressed and understood by both partners, often leads to divorce. Unfortunately, if the pattern is not recognized and resolved it re-emerges in second marriages and later intimate relationships.

Do you want to know how your relationship is doing? Take a relationship evaluation quiz here. If you are struggling with your relationship, don't wait to reach out for help.

What Does the Pursue-Withdraw Pattern Look Like?

This type of pattern is where one partner needs and seeks more closeness than the other. It's very destructive, and if not addressed carefully by them, it might lead to divorce.

Typically, withdrawers operate under the assumption that if they allow themselves to be vulnerable and assertively "put themselves out there" their partner will not validate their feelings and, at worst, they will leave. In order to maintain the relationship, they withdraw and shut down.

When the withdrawer does this, they ignore their own needs for emotional connection and closeness. They become consumed with feelings of hurt and resentment.

When this happen, the pursuer typically works harder to re-establish the connection. Rather than ignoring their own needs, the pursuer ramps up their efforts to "fix" the situation and reconnect to their partner.

The result of this pattern can be persistent fights, hurt feelings, andmisunderstandings. Overtime, erosionoftrust begins tooccur. Both partners endupfeelingunloved and abandoned.

UNDERSTANDING THE UNDERLYING ISSUES IN YOUR RELATIONSHIP

Every person has needs for emotional connection and security. We all long to feel loved, cared for, respected, and valued. When a pursue-withdraw pattern exists in a relationship for a longtime, it can be difficult to establish a sense of security. As time goes on, one or both partners beg into feel isolated and alone.

At this point, often the pursuer themselves becomes withdrawn. They feel hopeless and ready to move on. This is usually when the withdrawer understands something has changed, and the decision is made to either get a divorce or try therapy.

This is an unfortunate situation, because if you wait until the relationship gets to this point it can be extremely challenging to repair the hurt and restore trust.

Change the Pattern Before it Destroys your Relationship

If you understand that there is a repeating pattern of pursue-withdraw between you and your partner and you want to save the relationship, it is imperative that you both take steps to find a way to discover the underlying issues and work to resolve them. If divorce occurs, the pattern usually persists into second marriages.

It is essential to understand this pattern, what underlies it, and what is driving the behavioral reactions of each of you. When this understanding occurs, it is easier to meet the fundamental needs of each person in the relationship.

Have you ever fantasized about being with the partner of your dreams? If so, then you have already tapped into the tool that can help you actualize this in real life. Visualization, the kind that involves imagining success in love, has long been employed by professional athletes to create amazing results. Research is showing that many professions are already using thetools of visualization quiteeffectively – surgeons use it to possess laser focus; musicians use it to improve their performance; and business executives use it to ace a presentation. Many use it to stay on their diets to lose weight. You too, you can use visualization to call in your beloved and to experience the relationship you've always dreamed of.

TECHNIQUE 2: CULTIVATE SELF-COMPASSION

If you were to go on a journey with someone for several decades, how important would the relationship between the two of you be?

Wouldn't you make an effort to ensure you got along well? Wouldn't you want to make sure the relationship between the two of you was positive and supportive?

The journey of life, the one we're all on right now, isn't so different from that hypothetical journey. Except rather than spending time with another person, our constant companion is the voice inside our heads. But for many of us, the relationship between ourselves and that voice isn't so positive.

"You can search throughout the entire universe for someone who is more deserving of your love and affection than you are yourself, and that person is not to be found any where. You yourself, as much as anybody in the entire universe deserve your love and affection."- Buddha

AN INTRODUCTION TO SELF-COMPASSION

Rather than trying to change our deeply rooted values–a challenging task– we can start by lessening the impact they have on us by changing the ways in which we view ourselves. We can begin to do this with self-compassion.

Self-compassion means being gentle, kind and understanding with yourself; accepting that you are not perfect; and understanding that there is potential for learning and growth in every mistake you make.

If you don't love yourself, you cannot love others. You will not be able to love others. If you have no compassion for yourself then you are not able of developing compassion for others.

The Buddhist understanding of compassion means offering patience, kindness, and non-judgmental understanding to others as well as oneself. Contrary to what you might believe, self-compassion is not equivalent to selfishness.

An easy way to understand self-compassion is to compare it to the instructions given by flight attendants in case of a depressurized airplane cabin: you're supposed to put on your own oxygen mask before helping someone else with theirs. In the same way, we need to look after ourselves before taking care of others.

Make Peace with Your Inner Critic

People generally try to hide their shortcomings in order to maintain a positive self-image. With self-compassion, people can actually increase their knowledge and clarity about their own limitations

It might seem like that could end in a downward spiral, but self-compassion has been found to be positively correlated with improved mental health and greater life satisfaction.

So what can you do to turn our inner critic into a gentle supporter? Traditional cognitive skills training has been found rather ineffective in this area.

5 WAYS TO PRACTICE SELF-COMPASSION

Here are five essential steps to increase yourself-compassion using internal and external resources:

Step 1: Practice Forgiveness

Stop punishing yourself for your mistakes. Accept that you are not perfect and be gentle with yourself when you are confronted with your shortcomings. You are valued by your friends and colleagues because of who you are, not because you are faultless.

Become aware of times when you derive a sense of self-worth from performance or perfection. Understand that you do not need to be a certain way to be worthy of love.

One way to remind yourself that you are worthy, even when you're not performing well, is to put a sticky note near your desk or in your wallet with a message reminding you to be gentle and kind with yourself.

There is no sense in punishing your future for the mistakes of your past. Forgive yourself, grow from it, and then let it go.

Step 2: Employ a Growth Mindset

Do you view challenges as impossible obstacles or as opportunities to grow? Employing a growth mindset ismorehelpful.

Embrace rather than avoid challenges, persist in finding meaning in them, and don't give up on yourself. When you find you are criticizing yourself and negatively comparing yourself with others, try to find inspiration in their successes and strengths instead of feeling threatened.

Step 3: Express Gratitude

Feeling gratitude is very powerful. Rather than wishing for what we do not have, there is strength in appreciating what we do have, right now. You can choose to write a gratitude journal or go for gratitude walks. By focusing on our blessings we employ a gentler inner voice and move the focus away from our shortcomings and outward to the world, with all its beauty.

Step 4: Find the Right Level of Generosity

Raj Raghunathan (2016) has identified three different reciprocity styles: giver, taker, and matcher. Givers are the most generous people, and generosity is a great way of employing compassion. However, givers can be both the most successful and least successful people, as they may fall into a pattern of selfless giving that ignores their own needs.

For generosity to work in favor of your well-being, it cannot be selfless. So, when being generous, make sure you are aware of your own needs before progressing. Then consciously choose the recipient of your generosity, the resources you have available, and your level of energy based on what will support your own well-being.

Also, have fun being generous. See the difference you make and do not forget to give back to yourself. Doing good for others makes us happy, but only if it does not reduce our own levels of well-being.

Here are some of the best ways I've found to cultivate self-compassion:

1. Transform Your Mindset

Sadly, it's often challenging to lift yourself up (particularly if you're feeling really low or ashamed), but if you want to create compassion for yourself, you have to change your mindset.

For me, self-compassion started with changing my thoughts. I started focusing on the fact that my behavior was bad, not me. Once I started labeling behavior (instead of myself as whole), I was able to be kinder to myself and open up my mind to the possibility that I could make changes.

2. Speak (And Think!) Kindly About Yourself

Hand in hand with the first step is speaking and thinking kindly about yourself. Your words are incredibly powerful, and if you continuously tell yourself you're unworthy, a mess, or unforgiveable, you'll soon start to believe it.

I did this for a long time, calling myself things like "crazy" or "out of control," but once I started changing my words, stopping myself every time I wanted to laugh off my behavior with a negative label, I began having more compassion for myself.

I was a person making bad choices, not a bad person. If you struggle with this step, imagine talking about yourself as you would talk about your best friend.

3. Forgive Yourself For Your Mistakes

Forgiveness is vital for self-compassion. We all make mistakes, but not all of us forgive ourselves for them. Depending on the mistake, this can be a very daunting task, but keep in mind that you cannot go back (no matter how badly you might want to), so the best thing to do is to choose forgiveness and forward motion.

Whenever I did something inappropriate, instead of shrugging it off or excusing my behavior, I started apologizing for it, both to others and to myself. Again, I focused on the fact that I wasn't bad; it was my behavior that was.

4. Spend Time Doing Things You Truly Enjoy

If you're struggling with shame, enjoying pleasurable activities can be seen as something you don't deserve. But each and everyone of us deserves to engage in joyful, uplifting, and exciting experiences.

Allowing yourself to experience true happiness—to take time from your life to do something you love—is an act of compassion.

When I found myself feeling ashamed for a mistake I'd made, I began making a conscious effort to understand what situation provoked that act and I strive to make choices that put me in more positive situations.

5. Strive to Avoid Judgments and Assumptions

Though assumptions and judgments are often based on experience or knowledge of some sort, it's very hard to predict what will happen in life. When you judge yourself or make an assumption about what you will do in the future, you don't give yourself an opportunity to choose a different path. Instead of limiting yourself, be open to all possibilities.

In my situation, I started assuming that I shouldn't go to an event because I would inevitably cause a scene and have to leave. Little did I know that I'd eventually learn, with the help of therapy and self-compassion, to socialize. I had assumed that I would always be "wild," but I've learned that you cannot know the future. Assumptions will only inhibit you.

6. Find Common Ground with Others

While self-compassion is about the way you care for yourself, one of the best ways to cultivate it is to create connections with others. When you open yourself up to sharing who you are with others, you'll soon see that you're not alone.

We all struggle to treat ourselves with kindness, and recognizing this can make the struggle more manageable.

At some point, I began admitting to friends and family that I had a problem. It was difficult to open up emotionally, but the more I did, the more I discovered that I wasn't alone. Creating these stronger emotionalties made it so much easier to deal with my personal shame and to work toward more self-compassion.

7. Take Care of Your Mind and Your Body

One of the most compassionate things you can do for yourself is take care of your mind and body. Spend as much time as possible absorbing new information, and be sure to fill your mind and body with positive things (healthy food, good conversations, wisdom, etc.). Being mindful of what you consume and what you do with your energy is an important part of self-compassion.

Once I began doing this, I was able to recognize what did and didn't make me feel good about myself. Admittedly, I didn't always continue to seek out positive things (and still struggle to do so attimes), but the awareness of what would and wouldn't impact my mind and body positively gave me the opportunity to make more conscious, compassionate choices for myself.

"Self-care" is a trendy phrase these days, but what exactly does it means? Look on social media or in a magazine, and it might seem like the concept of self-care is just an excuse to indulge in luxury or to treat yourself in some way. But there's much more to it than that.

Self-care is the practice of asking yourself what you need – mentally, spiritually, or emotionally – and making sure you get it. It is not inherently indulgent or selfish; it is necessary. As adults, we are solely responsible for managing our own health, emotions, and personal growth. Self-care is the set of practices that allow us to accomplish this.

WHY SELF-CARE?

As flight attendants say, "Put on your own oxygen mask before assisting others." This cautionary instruction is a great self-care metaphor. Modern living makes it easy to overlook your own well-being in order to keep up with other responsibilities, but it's unsustainable and even risky to do so for the long term.

Maybe you've experienced one of these common symptoms of not taking enough care of yourself:

Compassion fatigue. - The kind of exhaustion that hurts your ability to experience joy and genuine care for others. When you're physically, mentally, emotionally, or spiritually drained, it's impossible to expend energy to be grateful and fully present for your loved ones. Compassion fatigue is like tryingto pour from an empty cup.

Burnout - A state of chronic stress from being overworked. Burnout is often career-related but it may also stem from school, family life, or any other type of occupation. Symptoms include physical and mental exhaustion, feelings of cynicism, irritability, or rigidity, and various states of "inoperability" – feeling ineffective, detached, or useless. Burnout often leads to unhealthy self-medication.

Poor physical health - Everything from doctors' appointments, to preparing healthy meals, to exercise and fitness classes count as physical self-care. Overlook these practices and you'll eventually experience an avoidable decline. Furthermore, a lack of self-care leads to increased stress, which has physically damaging effects of its own. Stress contributes to obesity, high blood pressure, heart disease, diabetes, and more.

The first step in quality self-care is to learn what it is and understand its importance. So if you're reading this article, congratulations! You're already on your way.

The next step is to believe that you deserve it, which is easier said than done. We repeat: taking timeout for yourself does not make you selfish, weak, or inferior in anyway! Only you have the power to manage your life. It's your responsibility to take good care of yourself. And, as we like to remind you, you deserve to feel better.

Part of this process is learning to silence the inner critic – the little voice in your head saying "It's not worth it", "You should be doing more," or "Everyone else is doing better". These critical, judgmental, self-blaming phrases reinforce the message that you're not enough and keep you feeling small and unworthy. So challenge this voice and realize it's not true. It's just a feeling. When you find yourself making the occasional unhealthy decision, don't beat yourself up about it. Be kind to yourself, forgive yourself, and plan how you'll do better next time.

If you want to take better care of yourself but don't know what to prioritize, try a self-exploration or reflection exercise to identify where you have the most to gain.

Long ago, I used to be ungrateful for what I had. I never actually realized the importance of gratitude until one day everything was taken from me and I found myself penniless, friendless and utterly hopeless. I learned a lot about the importance of having gratitude during that period in my life.

However, it's easy to be ungrateful these days, isn't it? It's easy to want things that we don't have. In fact, I'd even go so far as saying that it's stitched into the very fabric of our society. Consumer is misbaked right in. Everywhere we turn, we're reminded of the fact of how little we do have rather than how much we have to be grateful for.

In a society that's governed by the haves versus the have-nots, where money is all-powerful and helps epitomize the alluring facets of life like freedom, security and power, it's easy to be ungrateful. When you're working tirelessly to no avail, unable to get ahead in life, especially after enduring the heartache of failure or financial turmoil, it's simple to get delusional and it's easy to not be grateful.

If you find yourself in that situation right now, fear not, we've all been there. Yet, there are ways we can become grateful for the things we have in our lives. In fact, gratitude is quite possibly the most direct path way to success. The problem? Most people hinge their happiness and gratitude on achievement rather than making it a platform for such.

Recently I asked myself the question: "Why is it to so important to have gratitude in life?" Quite literally, what I realized over time, was that gratitude transformed my life. But I wasn't able to see all the things that I had to be grateful for until I experienced what I would call, monumental failures in life. The lessons gleaned from those failures were paramount for me.

Failure helps to instill the importance of gratitude. It allowed me to look at things differently, to see everything in a new light, with a new perspective. If you've failed at something, or you're living a lifeless than you feel you deserve, keep the faith. Keep up the hope because there's light at the other end of the tunnel.

What I've come to realize is that no matter the state or quality of our lives, whatever outcomes we've produced, goals we've reached (or failed to reach), what decisions we've made, and where we've ended up, has almost everything to do with focus. While some things might be out of our control, much of what happens based on our thoughts, emotions and behaviors, are largely a conditional response to our focus.

That's also why its so important to be grateful no matter what's happening in your life. Even if you're going through turmoil, and even if your entire world is crashing down around you, you have to be grateful. While it might sound strange, gratitude is the surest pathway to both success and happiness.

Whatever realm of thought you're living in, the importance of gratitude cannot be underestimated. There are specific reasons why gratitude can change your life, and if you listen to them and truly hear the message beyond the words, there are some incredible things that will begin to happen for you over time.

I'm a real-world testament to the truth in all of this — a living, breathing example of how gratitude can shift your life, creating monumental results. But don't just take it from me. Some of the most successful people in the world live by this school of thought. They believe, deep down inside, that the pathway to success, whatever definition that might take on for you, is through an ever-grateful attitude for what you have today, right now, in this very moment, rather than what you're lacking.

How to Practice Self-Care

- Develop a regular sleeping routine
- Aim for a healthy lunch
- Take lunch breaks
- Keep a reflex journal
- Engage in a non-work hobby
- Develop supportive friendships
- Go to see a movie or do something else you enjoy

- Go on bush walks
- Do yoga
- Reflect with a close friend or support

TECHNIQUE 3: DEVELOP SELF-AWARENESS

Self-awareness theory is based on the idea that you are not your thoughts, but the entity observing your thoughts; you are the thinker, separate and apart from your thoughts (Duval&Wicklund, 1972).

We can go about our day without giving our inner self any extra thought, merely thinking and feeling and acting as we will; however, we also can focus our attention on that inner self, an ability that Duval and Wicklund (1972) termed "self-evaluation."

When we engage in self-evaluation, we can give some thought to whether we are thinking and feeling and acting as we "should" or following our standards and values. This is referred to as comparing against our standards of correctness. We do this daily, using these standards as a way to judge the rightness of our thoughts and behaviors.

Using these standards is a major component of practicing self-control, as we evaluate and determine whether we are making the right choices to achieve our goals.

Our actions will also depend on how much time and effort we believe that alignment will take; the slower progress will be, the less likely we are to take on there alignment efforts, especially if the perceived discrepancy between ourselves and our standards is large.

Essentially, this means that when faced with a significant discrepancy that will take a lot of consistent and focused work, we often simply don't bother and stick to avoiding self-evaluation on this particular discrepancy.

Further, our level of self-awareness interacts with the likelihood of success in realigning ourselves and our standards to determine how we think about the outcome. When we are self-aware and believe there is a high chance of success, we are generally quick to attribute that success or failure to our efforts.

Conversely, when we are self-aware but believe there is a low chance of success, we tend to think that the outcome is more influenced by external factors than our efforts (Silvia&Duval, 2001). Of course, sometimes our success in realignment with our standards is driven in part by external factors, but we always have a role to play in our successes and failures.

Interestingly, we also have some control over our standards, such that we may alter our standards if we find that we don't measure up to them.

This is more likely to happen if we're focused more on the standards than on ourselves; if we fail when we are focused on the standards more than our performance, we are more likely to blame the standards and alter them to fit our performance.

Although it may sound like merely shifting the blame to standards and, therefore, letting yourself off the hook for a real discrepancy, there are many situations in which the standards are overly strict. Therapists' offices are filled with people who hold themselves to impossibly high standards, effectively giving themselves no chance of success when comparing themselves to their internal standards.

Its clear from the research on self-awareness that it is an important factor in how we think, feel, act, and react to our thoughts, feelings, and actions.

4 PROVEN BENEFITS OF SELF-AWARENESS

Now, let's shift our attention to research on the outcomes of being self-aware.

As you might imagine, there are many benefits to practicing self-awareness:

1. It can make us more proactive, boost our acceptance, and encourage positive self-development.
2. Self-awareness allows us to see things from the perspective of others, practice self-control, work creatively and productively, and experience pride in ourselves and our work as well as general self-esteem.

3. It leads to better decision making.
4. It can make us better at our jobs, better communicators in the workplace, and enhance our self-confidence and job-related wellbeing.

These benefits are reason enough to work on improving self-awareness, but this list is by no means exhaustive. Self-awareness has the potential to enhance virtually every experience you have, as it's a tool and a practice that can be used anywhere, anytime, to ground yourself in the moment, realistically evaluate yourself and the situation, and help you make good choices.

EXAMPLES OF SELF-AWARENESS SKILL

So we know that self-awareness is good, but what does it look like? How does one practice self-awareness?

Below are three examples of someone practicing self-awareness skills:

Bob at Work

Bob struggles with creating a quarterly report at work, and he frequently produces subpar results. He notices the discrepancy between his standards and performance and engages in self-evaluation to determine where it comes from and how to improve.

He asks himself what makes the task so hard for him, and he realizes that he never seems to have trouble doing the work that goes into the report, but rather, writing it up cohesively and clearly.

Bob decides to fix the discrepancy by taking a course to improve his writing ability, having a colleague review his report before submitting it, and creating a re-usable template for future reports so he is sure to include all relevant information.

Monique at Home

Monique is having relationship problems with her boyfriend, Luis. She thinks Luis takes her for granted and doesn't tell her he loves her or share affection enough. They fight about this frequently.

Suddenly, she realizes that she may be contributing to the problem. She looks inward and sees that she doesn't show Luis appreciation very often, overlooking the nice things he does around the house for her and little physical touches that show his affection.

Monique considers her thought processes when Luis misses an opportunity to make her feel loved and notes that she assumes he purposely avoids doing things that she likes. She spends time thinking and talking with Luis about how they want to show and receive love, and they begin to work on improving their relationship.

Bridget on her Own

Bridget struggles with low self-esteem, which causes depressive symptoms. She doesn't feel good enough, and she doesn't accept opportunities that come her way because of it. She begins working with a therapist to help her build self-awareness.

The next time an opportunity comes her way, she thinks she doesn't want to do it and initially decides to turn it down. Later, with the help of some self-awareness techniques, Bridget realizes that she is only telling herself she doesn't want to do it because of her fear that she won't be good enough.

Bridget reminds herself that she is good enough and redirects her thoughts to "what if I succeed?" instead of "what if I fail?" She accepts the opportunity and continues to use self-awareness and self-love to improve her chances of success.

These three stories exemplify what self-awareness can look like and what it can do for you when you tap into it. Without self-awareness, Bob would have kept turning in bad reports, Monique would have continued in an unsatisfying relationship or broken things off, and Bridget would never have taken the opportunity that helped her grow.

If you look for them, you can find these stories everywhere.

3 WAYS TO CULTIVATE SELF-AWARENESS

Now we have some clear cut examples of self-awareness in mind. We know what it looks like to embrace self-awareness and grow. But how do you do it? What did our leading characters do to practice self-awareness?

There are many ways to build and practice self-awareness, but here are some of the most effective:

1. Practice Mindfulness and Meditation

Mindfulness refers to being present in the moment and paying attention to yourself and your surroundings rather than getting lost in thought or ruminating or daydreaming.

Meditation is the practice of focusing your attention on one thing, such as your breath, a mantra, or a feeling, and letting your thoughts drift by instead of holding on to them.

Both practices can help you become more aware of your internal state and your reactions to things. They can also help you identify your thoughts and feelings and keep from getting so caught up in them that you lose your hold on your "self."

2. Practice Yoga

Yoga is a physical practice, but it's just as much a mental practice. While your body is stretching and bending and flexing, your mind is learning discipline, self-acceptance, and awareness. You become more aware of your body and all the feelings that manifest, and you become more aware of your mind and the thoughts that crop up.

You can even pair yoga with mindfulness or meditation to boost yourself-awareness.

3. Make Time to Reflect

Reflecting can be done in multiple ways (including journaling; see the next tip) and is customizable to the person reflecting, but the important thing is to go over your thoughts, feelings, and behaviors to see where you met your standards, where you failed them, and where you could improve.

You can also reflect on your standards themselves to see if they are good ones for you to hold yourself to. You can try writing in a journal, talking out loud, or simply sitting quietly and thinking, whatever helps you to reflect on yourself.

BODY LANGUAGE

From our facial expressions to our body movements, the things we don't say can still convey volumes of information.

It has been suggested that body language may account for between 60 to 65% of all communication. Understanding body language is important, but it is also essential to pay attention to other cues such as context. In many cases, you should look at signals as a group rather than focusing on a single action.

Here's what to look for when you'retrying to interpret body language.

Think for a moment about how much a person is able to convey with just a facial expression. A smile can indicate approval or happiness. A frown can signal disapproval or unhappiness.

In some cases, our facial expressions may reveal our true feelings about a particular situation. While you say that you are feeling fine, the look on your face may tell people otherwise.

Just a few examples ofemotions that can be expressed via facial expressions include:

- Happiness
- Sadness
- Anger
- Surprise
- Disgust
- Fear
- Confusion

- Excitement
- Desire
- Contempt

The expression on a person's face can even help determine if we trust or believe what the individual is saying. One study found that the most trustworthy facial expression involved a slight raise of the eyebrows and a slight smile. This expression, the researchers suggested, conveys both friendliness and confidence.

Facial expressions are also among the most universal forms of body language. The expressions used to convey fear, anger, sadness, and happiness are similar throughout the world.

Researcher Paul Ekman has found support for the universality of a variety of facial expressions tied to particular emotions including joy, anger, fear, surprise, and sadness.

Research even suggests that we make judgments about people's intelligence based upon their faces and expressions.

One study found that individuals who had narrower faces and more prominent noses were more likely to be perceived as intelligent. People with smiling, joyful expression were also judged as being more intelligent than those with angry expressions.

The Eyes

The eyes are frequently referred to as the "windows to the soul" since they are capable of revealing a great deal about what a person is feeling or thinking.

As you engage in conversation with another person, taking note of the movement of the eye is a natural and important part of the communication process.

Some common things you may notice include whether people are making direct eye contact or averting their gaze, how much they are blinking, or if their pupils are dilated.

When evaluating body language, pay attention to the following eye signals.

Eye Gaze. When a person looks directly into your eyes while having a conversation, it indicates that they are interested and paying attention. However, prolonged eye contact can feel threatening.

On the other hand, breaking eye contact and frequently looking away might indicate that the person is distracted, uncomfortable, or trying to conceal his or her real feelings.

Blinking: Blinking is natural, but you should also pay attention to whether a person is blinking too much or too little.

People often blink more rapidly when they are feeling distressed or uncomfortable. In frequent blinking may indicate that a person is intentionally trying to control his or her eye movements.

For example, a poker player might blink less frequently because he is purposely trying to appear unexcited about the hand he was dealt.

Pupil Size: Size of pupil can be a very subtle non-verbal communication signal. While light levels in the environment control pupil dilation, sometimes emotions can also cause small changes in pupil size.

For example, you may have heard the phrase "bedroom eyes" used to describe the look someone gives when they are attracted to an other person. Highly dilated eyes, for example, can indicate that a person is interested or even aroused.

The Mouth

Mouth expressions and movements can also be essential in reading body language. For example, chewing on the bottom lip may indicate that the individual is experiencing feelings of worry, fear, or insecurity.

Covering the mouth maybe an effort to be polite if the person is yawning or coughing, but it may also be an attempt to cover up a frown of disapproval.

Smiling is perhaps one of the greatest body language signals, but smiles can also be interpreted in many ways.

A smile maybe genuine, or it may beused to express false happiness, sarcasm, or even cynicism.

When evaluating body language, pay attention to the following mouth and lip signals:

Pursed lips: Tightening the lips might be an indicator of distaste, disapproval, or distrust.

Lip biting. People sometimes bite their lips when they are worried, anxious, or stressed.

Covering the mouth: When people want to hide an emotional reaction, they might cover their mouths in order to avoid displaying smiles or smirks.

Turned up or down: Slight changes in the mouth can also be subtle indicators of what a person is feeling. When the mouth is slightly turned up, it might mean that the person is feeling happy or optimistic. On the other hand, a slightly down-turned mouth can be an indicator of sadness, disapproval, or even an outright grimace.

Gestures

Gestures can be some of the most direct and obvious body language signals. Waving, pointing, and using the fingers to indicate numerical amounts are all very common and easy to understand gestures.

Some gestures may be cultural, however, so giving a thumbs-up or a peace sign in another country might have a completely different meaning than it does in the United States.

The following examples are just a few common gestures and their possible meanings:

A clenched fist can indicate anger in some situations or solidarity in others.

A thumbs up and thumbs down are often used as gestures of approval and disapproval.

The "okay" gesture, made by touching together the thumb and index finger in a circle while extending the other three fingers can be used to mean "okay" or "all right." In some parts of Europe, however, the same signal is used to imply you are nothing. In some South American countries, the symbol is actually a vulgar gesture.

The V sign, created by lifting the index and middle finger and separating them to create a V-shape, means peace or victory in some countries. In the United Kingdom and Australia, the symbol takes on an offensive meaning when the back of the hand is facing outward.

The Arms and Legs

The arms and legs can also be useful in conveying non-verbal information. Crossing the arms can indicate defensiveness. Crossing legs away from another person may indicate dislike or discomfort with that individual.

Other subtle signals such as expanding the arms widely may be an attempt to seem larger or more commanding while keeping the arms close to the body may be an effort to minimize one self or withdraw from attention.

When you are evaluating body language, pay attention to some of the following signals that the arms and legs may convey:

Crossed arms might indicate that a person feels defensive, self-protective, or closed-off.

Standing with hand splaced on the hips can be an indication that a person is ready and in control, or it can also possibly be a sign of aggressiveness.

Clasping the hands behind the back might indicate that a person is feeling bored, anxious, or even angry.

Rapidly tapping fingers or fidgeting can be a sign that a person is bored, impatient, or frustrated.

Crossed legs can indicate that a person is feeling closed off or in need of privacy.

Posture

How we hold our bodies can also serve as an important part of body language.

The term posture refers to how we hold our bodies as well as the overall physical form of an individual.

Posture can convey a wealth of information about how a person is feeling as well as hints about personality characteristics, such as whether a person is confident, open, or submissive.

Sitting upstraight, for example, may indicate that a person is focused and paying attention to what's going on. Sitting with the body hunched forward, on the other hand, can imply that the person is bored or indifferent.

When you are trying to read body language, try to notice some of the signals that a person's posture can send.

Open posture involves keeping the trunk of the body open and exposed. This type of posture indicates friendliness, openness, and willingness.

Closed posture involves hiding the trunk of the body often by hunching forward and keeping the arms and legs crossed. This type of posture can be an indicator of hostility, unfriendliness, and anxiety.

Personal Space

Have you ever heard someone refer to their need for personal space? Have you ever started to feel uncomfortable when someone stands just a little too close to you?

Intimate distance: 6 to 18 inches

This level of physical distance often indicates a closer relationship or greater comfort between individuals. It usually occurs during intimate contact such as hugging, whispering, or touching.

Personal distance: 1.5 to 4 feet

Physical distance at this level usually occurs between people who are family members or close friends. The closer the people can comfortably stand while interacting can be an indicator of the level of intimacy in their relationship.

Social distance: 4 to 12 feet.

This level of physical distance is often used with individuals who are acquaintances.

With someone you know fairly well, such as a co-worker you see several times a week, you might feel more comfortable interacting at a closer distance.

In cases where you do not know the other person well, such as a postal delivery only see once a month, a distance of 10 to 12 feet may feel more comfortable.

Public distance: 12 to 25 feet

Physical distance at this level is often used in public speaking situations. Talking in front of a class full of students or giving a presentation at work are good examples of such situations.

It is also important to note that the level of personal distance that individuals need to feel comfortable can vary from culture to culture.

One of t-cited example is the difference between people from Latin cultures and those from North America. People from Latin countries tend to feel more comfortable standing closer to one another as they interact while those from North America need more personal distance.

Understanding body language can go a long way toward helping you better communicate with others and interpreting what others might be trying to convey.

While it may be tempting to pick apart signals one by one, it's important to look at these non-verbal signals in relation to verbal communication, other non-verbal signals, and the situation.

You can also focus on learning more about how to improve your non-verbal communication to become better at letting people know what you are feeling—without even saying a word.

Your thoughts are an inner dialogue. You have an average of about six thousand thoughts a day, most of which you habitually repeat to yourself. In many cases, you learned to think these thoughts from experiences with your primary caregivers in childhood, and have been repeating them from that time.

Considering that cognitive abilities do not fully develop until the mid-20s, you can imagine how many of these thoughts no longer serve you.

Why develop your awareness of this inner dialogue? Your ability to choose how you think about yourself and lie around you allows you to regulate, or choose, your response to any triggering events.

Very simply, you want to become aware of what you tell yourself inside so that you rather than your emotions direct your choices. Your happiness depends on it. This is critical because your thoughts activate emotion-driven processes within you. That's right, even painful ones. Your thoughts, and the underlying beliefs that drive them, automatically trigger emotions.

While events and some people'sactions may trigger unpleasant feelings and reactions, they do not cause them. The real activating agents are what you tell yourself. And most of what you tell yourself operates subconsciously. It stems from the beliefs you hold at any given time, most ofwhich operate subconsciously.

When you, rather than your emotions, are in charge of what you think, you are in charge of your behaviors, and thus, have more say as to how events in your life unfold. Developing self-awareness is the first step to transforming your thoughts.

EMOTIONS

What is an Emotion

From a scientific point of view, an emotion is an intense and short-lived feeling caused by an evaluation of an (real or imagined) event that is of significant concern, and preparing the body to react or pay attention to the events. Regardless of which of emotion (e.g. anger, joy, sadness, etc.) you might experience, every emotion consists of five main components, where each have a distinct function.

Here are the 5 components that construct an emotion and their function:

1. **Cognitive** — Evaluate the event that leads to the emotion
2. **Neurophysiological** – Prepares your body to react to the event
3. **Motorexpression** – Expresses, or communicates your reaction to the event and how you will behave
4. **Motivational** – Prepares and directs your response toward the event

5. **Subjective feeling** – Monitors how your body feels in light of the event that is happening

Understanding When and Why Emotions Occur

Emotions play an important role in how we perceive and interact with our world. They can improve our lives for instance by:

- Letting us experience fear that stops us from doing potentially dangerous things (walking too close to the edge of a cliff)
- Making us experience happiness that reinforces newly made friendships
- Letting us experience anger that propels us to fight for causes that we care about

However, when emotions have the wrong intensity, duration, frequency, or type for a particular situation, they can also be very harmfultous. Think for instance of:

- Anger that lead us to hurt oneself or a loved one
- Fear of commitment that leads to broken relationships
- Anxiety that cripples your social and worklife

It is because of these unhelpful instances of emotions that it is beneficial to put effort into trying to control your emotions. Before we can try and exert this control, we first have to increase our emotional awareness, so that we will be more perceptive of the emotions that we are experiencing.

The first step in our journey to increase emotional awareness, is to take a closer look at what an emotion is exactly.

5 STEPS FOR IMPROVING YOUR EMOTIONAL INTELLIGENCE

Managing one emotion positively to relieve stress, communicating effectively, overcoming challenges, and stopping conflicts is crucial in a relationship. When building your emotional intelligence, you'll automatically sense the sensitivity that both of you are always seeking in a significant other through awareness.

Exercise 1: Past Emotional Event

To start off, think of the last time that you clearly felt an emotion. It doesn't matter which emotion you think of, as long as you have a clear (or as clear as possible) memory about the situation in which you experienced the emotion.

If you have a memory in your head, then we can start dissecting the situation and analyze it using these five components.

Step 1: The cognitive component of an emotion

The cognitive component of an emotion consists of the evaluation of the event that leads to the emotion. It is the "why" part of the emotion. So try and think back of the moment you experienced your emotion. Can you remember the event that caused it? Ask yourself:

- How was the event different from what you expected it to beat the moment?
- How likely was it that the event would bring you negative (or desirable) outcomes?
- How important was the event to your goals or needs at the time?
- Was the event caused by yourself, or by somebody else?
- Could the consequences of the event, at the time, have been avoided, or modified to your advantage?

Zoning in on the why of the situation will give you valuable information on what triggers these kinds of emotions for you. Knowing the trigger will increase your emotional awareness, as it will let you predict your future behavior, and how you might adjust your situation in order to elicit (or prevent) the (un)desirable emotion.

Step 2: The neurophysiological component of an emotion

Let's continue with the second component. The neurophysiological component of emotions are the bodily symptoms that you experience during emotions. It is the process your body starts in order to prepare you, or make you aware of the event that you are experiencing. Think back at how your body was acting when you experienced your specific emotion.

Were you:

- Getting pale, or blushing
- Feeling cold shivers, or feeling warm (pleasant)
- Heartbeat slowing down, or getting faster
- Breathing slowing down, or getting faster
- Muscles tensing, or relaxing

Not every body experiences emotions the same way. A good way to increase emotional awareness, is to try and determine for yourself which emotions are linked to which bodily reactions. Knowing the pattern of changes will increase the chance of accurately perceiving the emotion you are experiencing.

Step 3: The motor expression component of an emotion

Now let's take a look at the motor expression component of emotions. This component consists of the changes in facial and vocal expression, or bodily movements caused by the emotion. In otherwords, it is the way your body responds towards the event, in order to communicate or express how it's feeling at the time. Please try and think back on how your body language changed due to the event. Were you:

- Smiling, or frowning
- Moving towards, or withdrawing from people or things
- Moving abruptly, or freezing in one place
- Eyes opening, or closing
- Voice volume increasing, or decreasing
- Voice being assertive, or trembling

Similar to the previous component, knowing how you vocalize your emotion will not only help you increase your emotional awareness, but also give you insight into how you come across to other people. Do you for instance raise your voice when you are angry, or do you go quiet and stay silent in your anger. Once you know your behavior, you can ask yourself, "Is this the way I want to convey my anger". Knowing it will help you control your emotions, and help you refine your external behavior.

Step 4: The motivational component of an emotion

The next component is the motivational component of emotions. This component consists of the action you take in order to prepare and direct your attention toward the situation. Thinking back to your situation, did you:

- Move your attention towards, or away from the event
- Direct your attention towards yourself, or towards others
- Physically move yourself towards, or away from the event.

Awareness of your automatic behavior increases the possibility of adjusting this behavior towards behavior that is better suited for the situation.

Step 5: The subjective feeling component of an emotion

The subjective feeling component of emotions is the component that makes each emotional experience different from the other. Try and think:

- How intense was the emotion?
- How long did the emotion last?
- How good or bad was the emotion?
- How much arousal did the emotion bring forth?
- More importantly, try and think of why you experienced the emotion the way you did.
- Why was the emotion as intense as it was?
- Why did the emotion last as long as it did?
- Why was the emotion good or bad?
- Why was I so aroused by the emotion?

You can use this information to gauge how important an event is. Did you for instance get angrier than you expected when your coworker did not respect his deadline? Why do you think you got that angry? Or inversely, why didn't you get angrier? You can use your emotional awareness to reflect upon your emotions, which help you gauge how your current situation might hold up against your ideal situation.

Exercise 2: Upcoming Emotional Event

Now that we have dissected and analyzed a paste motion, it is time to push it up another level. As we've mentioned earlier, emotions are not only elicited by physical, or real situations, but also by imagined situations. The important part is that the situationis of great concerntous and is anchored in reality, meaning that it has a high likelihood of actually happening.

Think, for instance, of that important meeting you are going to have, or that big presentation that you have to give in front of the board of directors. It doesn't even have to be work-related. You might have that date with that cute girl, or guy, coming up, or meeting with the in-laws for the first time. It doesn't matter what the situation is, as long as it is important to you.

Let's do the same exercise again with an upcoming, important event. This time, instead of thinking about how you would feel, try and be aware of how you are feeling right now.

Following the same steps, we will first look at the cognitive component. Why is this event making you feel emotional?

- How was the event different from what you expected it to beat the moment?
- Is it likely that the event will bring you negative (or desirable) outcomes?
- How important is the event to your current goals or needs?
- Is the event caused by yourself, or by somebody else?
- Can the consequences of the event be avoided, or modified to your advantage?
- Next, let's try and really look at how your body is acting. Are you:
- Getting pale, or blushing
- Feeling cold shivers, or feeling warm (pleasant)
- Heartbeat slowing down, or getting faster
- Breathing slowing down, or getting faster
- Muscles tensing, or relaxing
- Depending on the importance of the situation, your bodily symptoms might be more prevalent.
- Lastly, how does this emotion feel at this time?

- How intense is the emotion?
- How long does the emotion last?
- How good or bad is the emotion?
- How much arousal does the emotion brings forth?

Emotional awareness will give your insight into how you are experiencing the emotion beforehand. Knowing how you will experience the emotion before hand, will help you gain control over the expression of your emotions in the future.

The more you do this exercise, the easier it gets. Therefore try to make it a daily routine to look back on the day and see if you can use these steps to dissect a situation.

HOW TO USE EMOTIONS TO YOUR ADVANTAGE

When people are aware of their own emotions, they are less likely to make judgment calls based on the emotions that they are experiencing at that particular moment.

For example, being happy can make you feel overconfident. Overconfidence may lead you to underestimate the risks of a situation, which can lead you to make a bad decision. On the other side, being sad can make you see things more negative than they actually are, therefore overestimating the risk of a situation, again leading to bad decisions.

Emotional awareness will guard you from this bias by improving your decision-making process. But do watch out, as being aware of your emotions is only half the fight.

Emotional awareness should therefore not only be used as an indicator about how you feel, but also as a tool that you must correctly use in your decision-making process.

Emotional awareness will not only benefit your judgment, but when vocalized, can also improve the quality of your relationship with your significant other.

Through the expression of positive emotions:

- Positive aspects of the relationship will be highlighted
- The perception of the relationship will improve

- The perception of you partner will improve
- This holds also true for the expression of negative emotions, as the expression of negative emotions:
- Provides important information on one's needs in a relationship
- Helps the significant other to respond in an appropriate and caring manner
- Expresses trust in the partner to show these negative emotions
- Increases support to work through these negative emotions

Most importantly, being aware of your emotions is the first step in gaining more control over your emotions. This is especially true for negative emotions, as awareness enables you to engage in repair behavior. It is therefore that higher emotional awareness is linked to lower social anxiety and depression.

In order to increase you emotional awareness you should try and make it a habit to analyze each emotional experience. So the next time, after you experience an emotion, try to dissect the situation using the five step method.

- What event happened that made me feel this emotion?
- What do I feel in my body?
- How did I express this emotion through my body language?
- What did I do in response of this emotion?
- How intense was the emotion?

First try and link your experience to specific emotions. Once you get better at recognizing single emotions, try and dissect a situation into multiple emotions.

In order to really improve, and make use of, your emotional awareness, try to make it a daily routine to scout ahead for upcoming emotional experiences. Using the same method:

- Why do you think you will experience this emotion?
- What do I feel in mybody?
- How intense is the emotion?

Practice makes perfect, and just as with any other skill, you need to put time and effort into it in order to improve your emotional awareness.

TECHNIQUE 4: INCREASE LOW SELF-ESTEEM

Self-esteem is how you feel about yourself, or the opinion you have about yourself. Everyone has times when they feel a bit low or find it hard to believe in themselves. However, if this becomes a long-term situation, this can lead to problems, including mental health issues such as depression or anxiety. Some of the symptoms of low self-esteem can also be a sign of these problems.

Not confident to stand for oneself or express your feelings, allowing yourself to become abused, belittle your partner on a constant basis, feeling attacked all the time, defensive all the time, can't even tell between constructive criticism and being bashed by harmful words, etc.

Self-esteem is often the result of a lifetime of experiences, and particularly what happened to us as children. However, it is possible to improve yourself-esteem at any age. This page provides more information about self-esteem, and some actions that you can take to improve it.

UNDERSTANDING SELF-ESTEEM

Some people think of self-esteem as their inner voice (or self-dialogue) – the voice that tells you whether you are good enough to do or achieve something.

Self-esteem is actually about how we value ourselves, and our perceptions about who we are and what we are capable of.

Self-Esteem is not About Ability

Self-esteem is often not associated with either your own ability, or other people's perceptions of you.

It is quite possible for someone who is good at something to have poor self-esteem. Conversely, someone who struggles with a particular task might generally have good self-esteem.

People with good self-esteem generally feel positive about themselves, and about life. This makes them much more resilient, and better able to cope with life's ups and downs.

Those with poor self-esteem, however, are often much more critical of themselves. They find it harder to bounce back from challenges and setbacks. This may lead them to avoid difficult situations. That can, however, actually decrease their self-esteem still further, because they feel even worse about themselves as a result.

A lack of self-esteem can therefore influence how people behave, not to mention what they achieve in their lives.

You may find it interesting to read our page The Importance of Mindset for more about how attitude influences behaviour.

Why Do People Experience Low Self-Esteem?

There are many reasons why someone might have low self-esteem. However, it often starts in childhood, perhaps with a feeling that you were unable to live up to expectations. It can also be the result of adult experiences such as a difficult relationship, either personal or at work.

Self-Esteem, Domestic Violence and Abuse

The victims of domestic violence and abuse often have low self-esteem.

This may be because their abuser has spent time belittling them and making them feel bad about themselves, reducing their self-esteem. However, it may also be that their low self-esteem made them more vulnerable to being abused because they did not feel that they were valuable.

Nobody should have to suffer from abuse or violence. If you, or anyone you know, is in this situation, you should seek help.

7 WAYS TO IMPROVE YOUR SELF-ESTEEM

There are a number of ways in which you can improve yourself-esteem.

1. Identify and Challenge Your Negative Beliefs

The first step is to identify, and then challenge, your negative beliefs about yourself.

Notice your thoughts about yourself. For example, you might find yourself thinking 'I'm not clever enough to do that' or 'I have no friends'. When you do, look for evidence that contradicts those statements. Write down both statement and evidence, and keep looking back at it to remind yourself that your negative beliefs about yourself are not true.

2. Identify the Positive About Yourself

It is also a good idea to write down positive things about yourself, such as being good at a sport, or nice things that people have said about you. When you start to feel low, look back at these things, and remind yourself that there is plenty of good about you.

In general, positive internal dialogue is a big part of improving your self-esteem.

If you catch yourself saying things like 'I'm not good enough' or 'I'm a failure', you can start to turn things around by saying 'I can be at this' and 'I can become more confident by viewing myself in a more positive way'.

To begin with you will catch yourself falling back in to old negative habits, but with regular effort you can start to feel more positive and build your self-esteem as well.

3. Build Positive Relationships—and Avoid Negative Ones

You will probably find that there are certain people—and certain relationships—that make you feel better than others.

If there are people who make you feel bad about yourself, try to avoid them.

Build relationships with people who make you feel good about yourself and avoid the relationships that drag you down.

4. Give Yourself a Break

You don't have to be perfect every hour of every day. You don't even have to feel good about yourself all the time.

Self-esteem varies from situation to situation, from day to day and hour to hour. Some people feel relaxed and positive with friends and colleagues, but uneasy and shy with strangers. Others may feel totally in command bof themselves at work but struggle socially (or viceversa).

Give yourself a break. We all have times when we feel a bit down or find it harder to maintain ourself-belief.

The key is not to be too hard on yourself. Be kind to yourself, and not too critical.

Avoid criticising yourself to others, because this can reinforce your negative views—and also give other people a (possibly false) negative opinion of you.

5. Become More Assertive and Learn to Say No

People with low self-esteem often find it hard to stand up for themselves or say no to others.

This means that they may become over-burdened at home or at work, because they do not like to refuse anyone anything. However, this can increase stress, and make it even harder to manage.

Developing your assertiveness can therefore help to improve yourself-esteem. Sometimes acting as if you believed in yourself can actually help to increase self-belief!

6. Improve Your Physical Health

It is much easier to feel good about ourselves when we are fit and healthy.

However, people with low self-esteem often neglect themselves, because they do not feel that they 'deserve' to be looked after.

Try taking more exercise, eating well, and getting enough sleep. It is also a good idea to make time to relax and to do something that you want to do, rather than something that someone else expects you to do. You may find that simple changes like this can make a huge difference to your overall outlook.

7. Take on Challenges

People with low self-esteem often avoid challenging and difficult situations.

One way to improve your self-esteem can actually be to take on a challenge. This doesn't mean that you need to do everything yourself—part of the challenge might be to seek help when you need it—but be prepared to try something that you know will be difficult to achieve.

By succeeding, you show yourself that you can achieve.

This challenges your negative beliefs and will therefore improve yourself-este.

CHAPTER 5: LIGHT UP YOUR RELATIONSHIP

TECHNIQUE 5: OVERCOMING OBSTACLES IN YOUR RELATIONSHIP TO EASE ANXIETY

Do you know the right questions to ask your significant other?

I mean, have you really, truly, deeply asked the best questions to get to know them as a person?

I'm a victim of the How Trap. The How Trap is when you are stuck only asking "How are you?" and nothing more. In the How Trap, you get caught up in day-to-day logistics and check-ins.

Put simply:

I don't want to know just how you are. I want to know who you are.

You know you are in the How Trap if:

Most of your questions start with "how." Like "how are you?" or "how are the kids?" or "how are you feeling?" or even, "how was your day?" These only touch the surface.

You don't make eye contact while you speak. You are doing the dishes, driving or cleaning up the house when you speak. This means your attention is not going deep.

You rely on social media posts to check-in. Do you feel like you already know everything that is going on in your people's lives because you follow them on social media? Sometimes this gets you caught in the how trap.

Sometimes we feel like we really know someone, but on the surface we are only familiar with the day-to-day. Psychology Professor Dan McAdams has studied what it takes to truly know someone. He believes there are "three levels of knowing" and that these are the three stages people progress through to become intimate friends, lovers, or companions.

Level 1 - General Traits at this level, you get to know someone's general personality traits. Specifically, where they fall on the Big 5 spectrum: how high or low they are in Openness, Conscientiousness, Extroversion, Agreeableness, and Neuroticism. See our overview of the personality traits here.

Level 2 - Personal Concerns This is where someone gets to know a person's goals, values, and motivations. They also get a broader picture of the decisions and attitudes that shape their life.

Level 3 - Self-Narrative Finally, when you truly know someone, you know the stories they tell themselves about themselves—how they have made sense of their journey and purpose through life.

The question is: *How do you move through these three levels?*

Level 1 is easy—typical conversation can help you with this.

Level 2 can happen naturally as you live with someone, travel with someone, and have shared experiences.

But Level 3 only can be done purposefully and with the right questions in a safe space. This brings me to the 36 couple questions.

THE 36 QUESTIONS

How to Ask the 36 Questions

Grab a Partner - Find your significant other, friend, parent, brother, sister, travel buddy, stranger you met online... really, ANYONE you want to get a little closer with! Make sure they are interested in completing the 36 questions with you.

Find Your Space - Find that quiet place where you won't be interrupted for at least 45 minutes to an hour. The last thing you want is to be interrupted by a phone call from your landlord!

READ: You do NOT have to do these all in one sitting—in fact, I recommend against it. Sometimes, intimacy takes time to build up. So start with one per dinner perhaps or one per car ride. Take your time, savor them, expand on them, and see where they take you. One of my friends and I answer one of these each week.

Focus on the Means Not the End - The questions are categorized in three different sets, with each set of questions a little bit more personal than the last. You'll take turns with your partner asking these questions, and both answering the questions.

It's important to NOT skip the questions, even if you know the answer to them. Keep in mind, vulnerability brings people closer. The point of these questions is to have sustained, escalating, and reciprocal self-disclosure. Take time having both people answer the questions and truly listen to the answers without judgment.

It'll look something like this:

Person A asks the first question.

Person B answers the first question.

Deep discussion! Aha moments! Surprises!

Person A answers the first question.

Deep discussion! Aha moments! Surprises!

Person B asks the second question.

And soon...

It's Not Polite to Stare

When you're finished asking the questions, there is ONE more step that the original experiment suggests:

Stare in your partner's eyes for four minutes.

This step is completely optional, but according to a 2019 study by Japanese researchers, eye contact activates the special parts of our brain responsible for empathy. If you really take the time to look into your partner's eyes, it'll be a special finish to your round of questions!

Just make sure to blink… otherwise, that's just a little bit creepy.

The 36 Questions

These 36 questions were developed by Aron A. et al (1997) www.landscape.com.au/live-love-lead-journal/36-qyestions-that-may-lead-to-love/ tohelp people breakthrough each of the intimacy levels. You can do these with your partner or with friends.

You can even print these out or email them to a friend!

Set 1 Questions

- *Given the choice of anyone in the world, whom would you want as a dinner guest?*
- *Would you like to be famous? In what way?*
- *Before making a phone call, do you ever rehearse what you're going to say? Why?*
- *What would constitute a perfect day for you?*
- *When did you last sing to yourself? To someone else?*
- *If you were able to live to the age of 90 and retain either the mind or body of a 30-year-old for the last 60 years of your life, which would you choose?*
- *Do you have a secret hunch about how you will die?*
- *Name three things you and your partner appear to have in common.*
- *For what in your life do you feel most grateful?*

- *If you could change anything about the way you were raised, what would it be?*
- *Take four minutes and tell your partner your life story in as much detail as possible.*
- *If you could wake up tomorrow having gained one quality or ability, what would it be?*

Set 2 Deep Questions

If a crystal ball could tell you the truth about yourself, your life, the future, or anything else, what would you want to know?

Is there something that you've dreamed of doing for a longtime? Why haven't you done it?

- *What is the greatest accomplishment of your life?*
- *What do you value most in a friendship?*
- *What is your most treasured memory?*
- *What is your most terrible memory?*
- *If you knew that in one year you would die suddenly, would you change anything about the way you are living now? Why?*
- *What does friendship mean to you?*
- *What roles do love and affection play in your life?*
- *Alternate sharing something you consider a positive characteristic of your partner. Share a total of five items.*
- *How close and warm is your family? Do you feel your childhood was happier than most other people's?*
- *How do you feel about your relationship with your mother?*

Set 3 Deeper Questions

Make three true "we" statements each. For instance, "we are both in this room feeling…"

Complete this sentence: "I wish I had someone with whom I could share…."

If you were going to become a close friend with your partner, please share what would be important for him or her to know.

Tell your partner what you like about them: Be honest this time, saying things that you might not say to someone you've just met.

- *Share with your partner an embarrassing moment in your life.*
- *When did you last cry in front of another person? By yourself?*
- *Tell your partner something that you like about them already.*
- *What, if anything, is too serious to be joked about?*
- *If you were to die this evening with no opportunity to communicate with anyone, what would you most regret not having told someone? Why haven't you told them yet?*
- *Your house, containing everything you own, catches fire. After saving your loved ones and pets, you have time to safely make a final dash to save any one item. What would it be? Why?*
- *Of all the people in your family, whose death would you find most disturbing? Why?*

Share a personal problem and ask your partner's advice on how he or she might handle it. Also, ask your partner to reflect back to you how you seem to be feeling about the problem you have chosen.

Do The 36 Questions Actually Work?

To find out if the questions actually work, let's turn to the creator of the 36 questions—a psychology professor named Arthur Aron.

Because there was a lack of love in the scientific community, Aron wondered: What's the best way to create love between two people?

So after numerous tests, he came up with these deliciously intimate questions to bring strangers closer together.

And when he put these 36 questions to the test, he found that…

Pairs of strangers who asked these 36 questions felt greater closeness than strangers who simply engaged in small talk.

How about couples in a long-term relationship? When I asked my husband these questions on a Friday date night, it was immediately a step-up from the usual "how was your day" spiel. We were both hooked as we fired off these questions back and forth! And the best part?

We both learned something new about each other.

That night, we finished dinner saying to each other, "Wow! I didn't know that about you!"

And we aren't the only ones that felt that way.

Before you work on learning how to improve communication in a relationship, you need to realize that not everyone has the same communication preferences. Some people like to talk, some prefer touch and others are more visual or respond better to gift giving than an outward discussion of feelings. You probably know which communication style you prefer, but what about your partner?

Communication and relationships are all different. Effective communication with your partner will come from acknowledging this. Your partner may be telling you exactly what they need, but you have to be cognizant of how they convey this information to you. If there's miscommunication, you'll miss the opportunity to build trust and intimacy, and you'll both feel frustrated.

When striving to learn how to communicate better, try watching your partner respond to different perceptive cues over a day or two. Does he or she seem to respond most to seeing and watching? Hearing and talking? Or touching and doing? For example, if your partner is more responsive to language, tone and other auditory cues, making lots of eye contact and gentle facial expressions may not be communicating as much to them as you think. You're sending signals but they're not picking them up. On the other hand, if you find that you are an auditory person and your partner is a kinesthetic person, remember that saying "I love you" may not be enough. Reinforce your love with touch, and remember to do so often.

KEYS TO COMMUNICATING IN RELATIONSHIPS

There are six fundamental needs that all humans share, but each of us puts these needs in a different order in accordance with our core values. Once you discover which needs matter the most to your partner, you'll know how to communicate with your partner and in a way that satisfies and fulfills them.

1. The first human need is the need for certainty. It's this need that drives us to seek out pleasure and avoid pain, stress and emotional

risks. Ask yourself these questions: How secure is my partner feeling in our relationship? We all find safety and comfort in different things. Be open with your partner about what gives them certainty and makes them feel stable.

2. The second human need that affects communication and relationships is the need for variety. Uncertainty isn't always scary if you know how to communicate with your partner. Relationships need healthy challenges that allow partners to grow together. As you learn how to communicate better, you'll find that variety keeps things fun and exciting with your partner.

3. Significance is the third human need: We all need to feel unique and important. Communication is key to this particular desire because your partner needs to know that you need them, in a singular way – that they fulfill your needs in ways that only they can. How do you demonstrate to your partner, not just tell them, that they are significant to you? You can show them through loving touch, offering them support when they need it and spending quality time with them.

4. The fourth basic human need is for connection and love. Every human needs to feel connected with others. Effective communication in relationships lets us know that we are loved and can make us feel at our most alive, but absence of love can cause pain like nothing else can. Too often we automatically say "I love you" in order to solve a conflict with our partners and forget to show love in a real, tangible way that speaks to our partner's needs. Reverse this pattern: Consciously show your partner that you love them every day, in a way that speaks to their personal preferences and needs. Learning how to improve communication in a relationship is about realizing what "language" your partner best understands and giving them love in that way.

5. Growth is the fifth human need. The human experience is one of motion and without constant growth, our relationships will become stale. We constantly endeavor to evolve along the different paths that interest us the most, whether these are emotional, intellectual, spiritual or otherwise. Your partner has the need for growth as much as you do and when we learn how to communicate better, wecan also learn how to better grow together. When was the last time you supported your partner's growth in

the areas that he or she is most passionate about? How can you continue to support them to the fullest?

6. The sixth and final human need is contribution and giving. Remember, the secret to living is giving. Contribution is our source of meaning – it determines who we become and solidifies our legacy, who we are and our role in the world. Consider what you give to your partner and how you can give more. Are you giving your time? Your undivided attention? The benefit of the doubt? A second chance? When communication in relationships is strong, both partners are able to continually come up with new and better ways of contributing to the other's happiness.

Determine if Your Partner's Needs are Being Met

There is one sure-fire way to know if your partner is getting these six human needs met in your relationship: ask her questions like; *when was the last time you thought about me in a positive way? What is your favorite thing that I do for you? What do you love about me? How supportive am I?* And then deeply listen to the answers. Reflect on what your partner says, and if you're not sure what he or she means, then ask by restating their point and asking if you understand correctly. The key to how to communicate in a relationship is often not in the actual verbal communication at all – it's in the way we listen to our partner.

Your partner may be communicating exactly what the problem is, but if you're not listening, you'll miss it. Resist the pull of just waiting for your partner to finish what they're saying so you can launch into your "turn." That isn't listening, it's waiting to talk. Instead, listen with a calm, open mind and really hear what they are saying to you. This will not only help you learn how to communicate better, but will also enable you to connect with your partner on a deeper level.

Be Honest and Open

Being honest and open should be at the top of the list for how to improve communication in a relationship. Say what you mean, and make your feelings and your needs clear. Retreating from conflict seems deceptively safe and comfortable, but it's no substitute for trust in a relationship and it will never help you learn how to communicate better. Walking away from an argument is a temporary way to deal with an on going communication issue and should only be done to achieve a brief cooling-down period. When you disagree with your partner, you must be able to trust that what you say will be heard and respected, and so does your partner.

If you or your partner (or both of you) is averse to conflict, you may find yourselves burying your emotions to please eachother and avoid problems. This temporary peace keeping band-aid turns a two-way relationship into a one-way street, and that's not a sustainable outcome. The happiness and intimacy you used to share will gradually erode, and it will take the relationship with it. Instead of ignoring issues, it's crucial that you both learn how to communicate better with each other.

Be Present in Your Relationship

To improve communication in relationships and truly understand what your partner is telling you, be present. Put time aside and dedicate yourself 100% to communicating with your partner. They should truly feel that they have your full attention and that they are your number one priority.

It's difficult to listen and be fully present, aware and mindful when you're angry and stressed or are working on things that take time away from your relationship. This is a part of life, but it's important to realize that it's not an excuse for neglecting communication in relationships. Remember that intimacy, love and trust are built when times are hard, not when they're easy. If we gave up at every sign of resistance, we would never progress band evolve. Seize these opportunities to learn how to deal with conflict and stress in a healthy manner and watch as you grow and flourish with your partner.

Let Things Go

Resist letting a simple discussion about what's happening now devolve into a rehash of every wrong that has ever happened between you and your partner. This is the opposite of loving and effective communication in relationships. Instead, assess the present situation and identify what you can do at this moment. Pause and remember why you're here, and remember that your goal, the outcome that you value, is to strengthen your relationship, build intimacy and learn how to communicate better. There's absolutely nothing either of you can do about the past right now, so let it go.

How to communicate better is about more than saying the right things. You should also be aware of your body language. You could offer all the loving and supportive words in the world to your partner, but if your arms are crossed over your chest and you have a scowl on your face, your partner is unlikely to respond favorably. How to communicate in a relationship means listening, loving and supporting with your whole being. Lean toward your partner, keep your face relaxed and open and touchthem in a gentle manner. Show them through ally our words, actions and expressions that you are their number one fan even if you are in conflict.

Break Negative Patterns

You know what your partner needs and have thought about their preferred communication style, but there's something else that affects communication in relationships: how you're speaking. Experts on communication break down the way we talk into pitch, pace, volume and timbre. The next time you're in a disagreement with your partner, be mindful and make conscious efforts to modulate these aspects of your voice.

- A voice that is overly high-pitched sounds defensive and immature. Also, if you end a sentence with a higher pitch, it sounds like a question; don't do this unless you're actually asking a question, or you may instill doubt in your partner.
- Pace just means how fast you're talking. Take a deep breath and slow down – especially when you're disagreeing. Speak calmly and clearly to get your message across.
- Pay attention to volume, especially volume "creep," and avoid competing to be heard – competition only leads to shouting and miscommunication. Being louder won't help you communicate with your partner. If your partner is speaking, you should listen.
- Timbre refers to your voice's emotional quality, attitude and tone. Pay careful attention to this, and watch for red flag timbres like

sarcasm that can erode communication in relationships and caused is trust between partners.

When things do get out of hand, break the pattern: Be playful and use humor in a way that keeps the conversation flowing in the right direction. Injecting humor into the situation can make it feels less dire and can yield amazing results for the two of you. That's because humor helps you regain perspective and balance; it is an essential component of healthy communication in relationships. It also relieves stress and improves your physical happiness in your everyday life. The biggest benefit to laughing in this context is that it reminds you that you love just being together with your partner. It reminds you that you can enjoy your time together, even when things seem challenging.

When learning how to communicate in a relationship, it's important to break the pattern of hostility, hurt and retreat. For example, when you catch yourself raising your voice or being sarcastic, change your tone. If you're using "you" repeatedly and blaming your partner, switch to "I" and "me," or better yet, "we." There's no point in off loading all your relationship's issues on to your partner. There are two people in every relationship, so don't shift the blame to be entirely on their shoulders.

Breaking the pattern is a powerful way of reframing the discussion and bringing it back to a level where you can get to what matters. Communication in relationships is all about what your partner's needs are, what your needs are and how you can both feel fulfilled from your relationship.

There are few things more damaging to a relationship than deceit. Many people believe trust either exists or it doesn't. In actuality trust is earned overtime and fragile once it exists. If it's broken, it can take a lot of time and work to rebuild. Despite that there are still people who seem to have a loose relationship with the truth and routinely hurt their partner and damage their relationship by lying.

If you are in a relationship with a person that you have a hard time trusting it can be nearly impossible to feel comfortably happy and secure. That doesn't mean you don't love them though. So, what can you do if you're dealing with deceit in your relationship and still love your partner?

DECEIT VS. LYING

Many assume that lying and deceit are the same thing when they actually aren't. Lying is a form of deceit, but deceit is the larger, over arching act of encouraging or allowing someone to believe something that isn't true. If you lie you are being deceitful but being deceitful doesn't always include lying. In fact, some of the most painful acts of deceit may not include outright lies at all.

Lying is the actual act of making untrue statements. Saying, "I didn't drink any beer last night" when you actually did is clearly lying. Cleaning up all evidence of the drinking and not owning up to it when your partner says, "I'm so happy you didn't drink any beer last night!" is being deceitful.

Although it's very common for lying and deceit to go hand-in-hand, they don't have to. Master manipulators, for instance, make a point of never overtly lying but use deceit in order to get what they want. Manipulators often imply things without stating them directly leaving victims thinking they heard something that was never actually said. This can lead to gas lighting and emotional abuse.

So, the first thing to do when you feel there is deceit in your relationship is to understand what it is you're honestly dealing with.

UNDERSTANDING THE REASONS FOR DECEITFUL BEHAVIOR

As with any problematic behavior, understanding why it's occurring is an important part of correcting it (or getting away from it if needed). Often, the reasons for behaviors are deeply embedded in a person's past experiences. In some cases, they may not even realize what they're doing or why it's wrong.

People lie for many reasons and some would argue that certain kinds of lies are okay, the little "white lies" for instance. These lies are often positioned as selfless and done to protect another person from being hurt.

Although a person may have good intentions, I don't agree with the idea there are acceptable lies. In my counseling experience lies and deceit are never really ultimately fort he benefit of someone else. They are selfish.

The reasons for lying typically fall into one of 4 categories.

1. To protect the person lying from experiencing discomfort.
2. To keep them from getting in trouble
3. To help them get something they want but haven't earned.
4. To allow them to get away with something they shouldn't be doing

That being said, the psychological motivation for being deceitful can vary. While some people are deceitful with intent to harm, others may believe they're behaving out of love.

Those who lie and deceive but feel truly convinced they are doing it for "good reasons" may have grown up in an environment where that behavior was common. They may not understand how to communicate in a truthful and honest manner because they were never taught. Or they felt the only way to protect themselves from pain was through lying.

Understanding the motivation for your partner's behavior, whatever it may be, doesn't make being deceitful acceptable. No matter how you slice it, lying and deceit damages trust and prevent shaving a healthy and happy relationship. And depending upon the motivation and what the deceit is covering up there can be even larger issues to contend with.

But behavior that isn't addressed doesn't get better on it's own, so you will need to find a way to begin the conversation. This can be tricky, because when dealing with deceit conversations can easily devolve into accusations, defensiveness, and addition allies very quickly. All of this can make it difficult to have a productive conversation regarding the damage the deceitful behavior is causing.

It can be much more productive to focus on creating a unified and clear goal to improve the general health of your relationship. Once you agree on that as the focus you can discuss the things that need to be done in order to achieve it – including the importance of honesty.

Depending upon your partner's history and reasons for the deceit, this is a process that may need to be repeated. It's also quite possible that true change will require the assistance of a professional counselor as the drivers for the behavior will need to change as well.

Regardless, change doesn't happen overnight and your patience will be required. But achieving that change is crucial since there is no way for a relationship with a deceitful partner to be a healthy, successful, or long-lasting one.

Watching out for these signs can help you head off a crisis and avoid disaster altogether. When you reach a point in a relationship when you think things might be getting serious, it is time to make an assessment of whether your prospective significant other is a deceptive person. The early stages of a relationship are mostly about fun, but you should keep an eye out for signs right from the get-go. Knowing what to look for will save you trouble and heartbreak in the future.

THE WARNING SIGNS

Secrecy - A bit of privacy in a relationship is important. It is healthy to maintain your own separate identity within the relationship, but when you or your significant other begins to hide details and important information from eachother, this is a sign that there is a lack of trust.

Obviously, keeping quiet about a surprise for your sweetheart is entirely different from something like lying about losing your job or how you feel about your partner's family.

Lies and Deception - One could argue that this is the daughter of the first warning sign. It certainly indicates a lack ofrespect. Lies and deception clearly do not happen in a healthy relationship.

Dependence and Control - Rare is the relationship that can function in a healthy fashion where co-dependency exists. Equally rare is the relationship that can function in a healthy fashion when one person is dominating the other. If you find these dynamics are at play, take a step back and look at them.

Fear - We all experience fear at various times in our lives. When it is persistent, it is important to examine the source and resolve it. Fear should not be a regular part of our relationships. If it is, it could be a sign of a larger problem.

There are various instances in life when a person experiences pain. This pain can be emotional, physical pain, or mental pain. Regardless of the nature of pain, it does have an impact on the person. Pain changes people. At that time, it is normal for a person to feel that life is pain. Experience teaches you eventually that with no pain, there is no gain. But as time passes, you learn to deal with your pain.

Pain breaks a person. But being broken is a privilege because a person whose hopes and dreams have been shattered or who has gone through immense pain in his life is more careful. Anxiety makes a person more durable and can also make someone weaker. It creates boundaries and also sets people free. Pain is powerful. Pain is an emotion everyone experiences in some form or the other in their lifetime.

Although we try, we cannot avoid pain altogether. Sometimes, grief comes in the most unexpected forms in our lives, and sometimes, it comes giving a prior signal. The fact is that pain changes people, sometimes in the right way and sometimes in the wrong direction. Pain is all in mind. Even physical pain has to felt in spirit. If the nerves of a damaged body area have been numbed, we will not feel the pain. The nerves send the signal to our brains to feel the pain. Our mind makes us feel pain.

But the best side effect of pain is that it makes people grow. They either grow and get stronger and learn to avoid future instances of pain, or they become more reliable and smarter and learn to deal with future cases of illness.

PAINFUL EVENTS OR OCCURRENCES IN LIFE

Pain occurs in our lives in many forms. These forms can be physical or emotional. Let us see what the different kinds of pain a human may experience, and its impact on their lives are.

Physical Pain - Hurt, pregnancy, disease, assault, or accident may result in physical pain. This kind of pain is felt by the person in the respective area of the body. Although the mind makes you feel physical pain too, you can relate this kind of a shock to that hurt or aching body area. The human body is very fragile. Any kind of forceful impact on the body in physical pain. This kind of pain often heals with time. It might leave scars in some cases, but the pain goes away. The memory might remain, but the feeling of sadness goes away.

This concept can also be taken lightly. As the pain saying goes, 'No pain, no gain,' it teaches us an essential fact in our day to day lives too. If you do not go through physical pain, you cannot get a fit body. Fitness for you can be achieved only after you dedicatedly go through some pain and effort.

Emotional Pain - The death of a loved one, relationship failures, failure in academics or career, financial conditions, fights, or unfair judgments is some instances when a person goes through emotional pain. The heart is deeply hurt, and the mind is frustrated and angry. This pain is equally burning, although it is not visible. This kind of pain is often more powerful in changing people than physical pain. A person who goes through emotional pain is privileged because they become more reliable and smarter to deal with similar instances in the future. If you wonder why memories are essential, then you should know that memories of past pain make you more robust and more careful in the future.

Can Pain Be Avoided?

Whether the pain can be avoided or not is entirely subjective. A child who burnt his hand playing with fire goes through immense pain. This pain teaches him to be careful with shooting the next time. He has learned his lesson and therefore avoids going through the same pain again.

Similarly, a lover hurt in love because of his partner's lack of loyalty is very careful before getting into a love relationship again. The earlier pain has taught him to think twice before committing himself to love again. The initial shock has him to be careful, and therefore he now avoids the same kind of pain.

But you cannot predict life and hence cannot predict pain. It can come in different ways without letting you know. The child who burnt his hand might avoid the pain from the fire the next time, but may fail at preventing the pain caused by a bad fall. Similarly, a lover hurt in love before might be careful in choosing a life partner the next time, but he cannot avoid the pain given to him by his friends or family.

Furthermore, there are certain kinds of pain that one has to experience in their life without avoiding. You cannot prevent the death of your loved ones, and you will have to go through immense pain when they pass away. Similarly, most women go through the pain of pregnancy and delivering a baby. They are aware of the pain, yet they want to experience it. Some kinds of pain have to be dealt with and experienced.

How Pain Changes People?

Trustless and be more guarded. Pain is an excellent teacher. In some cases, it teaches people to be more guarded and careful. A happy spirited girl who had a habit of making friends with everyone in school was often laughed at and made fun of by her peers. This caused her so much pain that she has now totally become an introvert. With no discomfort, she would have never learned to be more guarded and careful in life.

A little girl who was raped when she was out playing in the fields, got so scared that she stopped going out altogether. She became so guarded that she refused ever to let her guard down.

Pain makes people think that a similar danger is always lurking around them. They are always guarded.

Overthink more - Pain makes some people overthink more. They think of all the possibilities of a situation. They over think so much only to avoid further pain and hurt. They think of a case from all possible angles because they are more protective, careful, and guarded.

An investor who has incurred severe losses by investing in a project that failed now overthinks before re-investing. Pain, in this case, has made the person smarter and more experienced. He does not take to make investments easily now. He thinks and thinks and researches thoroughly before he reinvests.

Get more cautious and careful - Pain makes people more careful of their steps. It kills their free-spirits and makes them always cautious of the possible potholes ahead. Such people avoid taking chances or risks in life too.

A person who has been involved in a car accident before will now cautious in driving. Pain has changed the person for the better, and he is now more responsible and careful.

But in a similar incident, an investor who has lost a good deal of money in a past project now is scared to invest in anything lucrative again. Pain makes them avoid taking risks orchances in life.

Be more pessimistic: Pain also makes some people very negative and pessimistic. They always hoard negative opinions or thoughts about others. Nobody wants to bear such cynical people. Pain has changed them for the worse.

A person who has always failed in academics becomes a school dropout. Such people are very pessimistic with their kids too. Instead of appreciating their efforts, they only give negative comments. Such people ruin not only their happiness but also the joy of their children. Pain makes people cynical.

Tend to shut people off: Pain makes some people so scared of society that they completely shut themselves off. They forget to laugh, mingle, or share their feelings with the world at large. They feel that everyone is going to leave them. Such people tend to shut off from the world and keep struggling with their pain.

A person who has always been made fun of or being fat completely shuts himself from his friends, teachers, parents, and society. He now likes being alone and has no friends but deep inside his thoughts, he struggles with the feeling of being worthless.

There is no love without pain and there is no life without pain. Pain is how we gain our wisdom and our strength and it's how we develop thick skin. But in between pain and wisdom, we change — because no one gets out of pain the same person they used to be.

We still love. But with our guards up high, not as reachable as we used to be, not as trusting, not as innocent, not as pure and not the hopeless romantics we once were. We're cautious, we're afraid, we don't want to get rejected, we don't want to be bitter and we don't want to repeat the same mistakes again. We break hearts to save our own and we can live years without telling someone how we feel because we know they don't feel the same way.

We love, but we don't love wholeheartedly anymore, we love in pieces, we love when we're certain about someone's feeling and we love when the timing is on our side, we love only when it's safe.

We still hope but we also fear; we think of how things can go wrong, how good things will be short-lived, how things will not go the way we want them to because that's easier to handle, it's easier to deal with bad outcomes when you expected them. We live, but we don't completely give in to happiness, we don't believe that good things will last, we think that life will some how take it all back.

We don't give life a change to surprise us because we don't want to be disappointed again so we disappoint ourselves. We try to predict that life will let us down so when it does, we won't be broken.

We still dream. But we don't dream too big and we don't try to chase our dreams because we don't want to lose again, we don't want to fail, we don't want to feel like we're worthless. We want to prove that we're good enough, that we're capable of depending on ourselves, that we're responsible adults, so we dream within reach, we dream about what we know we can attain, we don't lookup, we don't look too far away and we don't believe in miracles. We dream, but we don't follow our dreams, we don't think they'll happen to us, we don't think we deserve that kind of happiness because we're used to pain.

We Stopped Believing in Miracles Ever Since Our Dreams Became Nightmares

- Pain changes people; mostly for the better, but when people suffer, they try to do everything they can to avoid it, they don't want their hearts to sink into the ground again, they don't want to cry uncontrollably again and they don't want to feel weak again.
- But when we try to avoid pain, we sometimes avoid pleasure. When we try to avoid pain, we avoid taking risks that could change our lives, when we try to avoid pain, we avoid loving and being loved in return.
- Sometimes I wish pain didn't change us, I wish pain didn't get so deeply to us so we can love, live, hope and dream like we used to. So we can believe in happiness and miracles the way we used to.

- Sometimes I wish we could change pain instead of pain changing us, so we can find a way to be ourselves again, to be the people we used to be before we were broken.
- Relationships can be deliciously breathtaking and at times ridiculously frustrating. It depends in part how we react or respond to relationship challenges. Here's a list of opportunities where relationships provide us the option to step in and grow, rather than resist and struggle.

Embrace change - Nature isn't stagnant and we'repart of nature. Don't expect things to be the way they were in the beginning because they won't ever be. But they can be better andricher.

Learn how to love deeply - Yourself and your partner. Your partner's role is not to make you happy. You WILL annoy each other. Learn how to love even when they aren't loveable.

Kick your ego to the curb - Instead of letting your mind and ego take the wheel, find ways to connect intimately. Feel into love and lead with your heart.

Accept imperfections - Life and relationships are messy. Instead of blaming your partner and focusing on what's wrong, look for the beauty and the positives.

Develop empathy - We all have hurts and empathy is hard when our ego wants to be heard. Put your ego on the shelf for a few moments, listen and feel your partner's experience.

Learn to fight fair - Own your anger without rage or shutting down. Even the happiest of couples argue. It's not that you DO argue – its how you argue and how youre solve things that matters.

Be a person of integrity - Yes, the old adage, "actions speak louder than words" is true so hold yourself accountable. Honor your word with your actions.

Choose positive over negative - Assume that your partner is doing the best they can in any moment based on what they're experiencing. Let go of negative mind chatter.

Step into vulnerability - It requires courage in making it a strength and not a weakness. Not being vulnerable is easy and an argument can be made that it's a weakness.

Build resilience - Know that things won't be all rainbows and orgasms. Learn what you need to nurture yourself and your spirit and do it often to build resilience.

Its very rare for couple not to run into a few bumps in the road. If you recognize ahead of time, though, what those relationship problems might be, you'll have a much better chance of getting past them.

Even though every relationship has its ups and downs, successful couples have learned how to manage the bumps and keep their love life going, says marriage and family therapist Mitch Temple, author of The Marriage Turn around. They hang in there, tackle problems, and learn how to work through the complex issues of everyday life. Many do this by reading self-help books and articles, attending seminars, going to counseling, observing other successful couples, or simply using trial and error.

HOW TO SOLVE THE MAIN 5 RELATIONSHIP PROBLEMS

1. Relationship Problem: Communication

All relationship problems stem from poor communication, according to Elaine Fantle Shimberg, author of Blending Families. "You can't communicate while you're checking your BlackBerry, watching TV, or flipping through the sports section," she says.

Problem-solving strategies:

- Make an actual appointment with each other. If you live together, put the cell phones on vibrate, put the kids to bed, and let voicemail pick up your calls.
- If you can't "communicate" without raising your voices, go to a public spot like the library, park, or restaurant where you'd be embarrassed if anyone saw you screaming.

- Set up some rules. Try not to interrupt until your partner is through speaking, or ban phrases such as "You always ..." or "You never ...."
- Use body language to show you're listening. Don't doodle, look at your watch, or pick at your nails. Nod so the other person knows you're getting the message and rephrase if you need to. For instance, say, "What I hear you saying is that you feel as though you have more chores at home, even though we're both working." If you're right, the other can confirm. If what the other person really meant was, "Hey, you're a slob and you create more work forme by having to pick up after you," they can say so, but in a nicer way.

2. Relationship Problem: Sex

Even partners who love each other can be a mismatched, sexually. But having sex is one of the last things you should give up. Sex brings us closer together, releases hormones that help our bodies both physically and mentally, and keeps the chemistry of a healthy couple healthy.

Problem-solving strategies:

- Plan, plan, plan. Fay suggests making an appointment, but not necessarily at night wheneveryone is tired. Maybe during the baby's saturday afternoon nap or a "before-work quickie." Ask friends or family to take the kids every other Friday night for a sleepover. "When sex is on the calendar, it increases your anticipation," Fay says. Changing things up a bit can make sex more fun, too, she says. Why not have sex in the kitchen? Or by the fire? Or standing up in the hallway?
- Learn what truly turns you and your partner on by each of you coming up with a personal "Sexy list," suggests California psychotherapist Allison Cohen. Swap the lists and use them to create more scenarios that turn you both on.
- If your sexual relationship problems can't be resolved on your own, Fay recommends consulting a qualified sex therapist to help you both address and resolve your issues.

3. Relationship Problem: Money

Money problems can start even before the wedding vows are exchanged. They can stem, for example, from the expenses of courtship or from the high cost of a wedding. The National Foundation for Credit Counseling (NFCC) recommends that couples who have money woes take a deep breath and have a serious conversation about finances.

Problem-solving strategies:

- Be honest about your current financial situation. If things have gone south, continuing thesamelifestyleisunrealistic.
- Don't approach the subject in the heat of battle. Instead, set aside a time that is convenient and non-threatening for both of you.
- Acknowledge that one partner may be a saver and one a spender, understand there are benefits to both, and agree to learn from each other's tendencies.
- Don't hide income or debt. Bring financial documents, including a recent credit report, pay stubs, bank statements, insurance policies, debts, and investments to the table.
- Don't blame.
- Construct a joint budget that includes savings.
- Decide which person would be responsible for paying the monthly bills.
- Allow each person to have independence by setting aside money to be spent at their discretion.
- Decide upon short-term and long-term goals: It's OK to have individual goals, but you should have family goals, too.
- Talk about caring for your parents as they age and how to appropriately plan for their financial needs if needed.

4. Relationship Problem: Conflict

Occasional conflict is a part of life but if you and your partner feel like you're starring in your own nightmare version of the movie Groundhog Day -- i.e.the same lousy situations keep repeating day after day -- its time to break free of this toxic routine. When you make the effort, you can lessen the anger and take a calm look at underlying issues.

Problem-solving strategies:

- You and your partner can learn to argue in a more civil, helpful manner. Make these strategies part of who you are in this relationship.
- Realize you are not a victim: It is your choice whether you react and how you react.
- Be honest with yourself: When you're in the midst of an argument, are your comments geared toward resolving the conflict, or are you looking for payback? If your comments are blaming and hurtful, it's best to take a deep breath and change your strategy.
- Change it up: If you continue to respond in the way that's brought you pain and unhappiness in the past, you can't expect a different result this time. Just one little shift can make a big difference. If you usually jump right in to defend yourself before your partner is finished speaking, hold off for a few moments. You'll be surprised at how such a small shift in tempo can change the whole tone of anargument.
- Give a little, get a lot: Apologize when you're wrong. Sure it's tough, but just try it and watch something wonderful happen.
- You can't control anyone else's behavior. "The only one in your charge is you."

5. Relationship Problem: Trust

Trust is a key part of a relationship. Do you see certain things that cause you not to trust your partner? Or do you have unresolved issues that prevent you from trusting others?

Problem-solving strategies:

- You and your partner can develop trust in each other by following these tips, Fay says.
- Be consistent.
- Be on time.
- Do what you say you will do.

- Don't lie – not even little white lies to your partner or to others.
- Be fair, even in an argument.
- Be sensitive to the other party feelings. You can still disagree, but don't discount how your partner is feeling.
- Call when you say you will.
- Call to say you'll be home late.
- Carry your fair share of the workload.
- Don't overreact when things go wrong.

THINGS TO DO TO MINIMIZE MARRIAGE PROBLEMS

Even though there are always going to be issues in a relationship you both can do things to minimize marriage problems if not avoid them altogether.

- First, be realistic. Thinking your mate will meet all your needs -- and will be able to figure them out without your asking -- is a Hollywood fantasy. Ask for what you need directly.
- Next, use humor – learn to let things go and enjoy one another more.
- Finally, be willing to work on your relationship and to truly look at what needs to be done. Don't think that things would be better with someone else. Unless you address problems, the same lack of skills that get in the way now will still be there and still cause problems no matter what relationship you're in.

A lot of us spend time daydreaming about things we wish we were doing in life, but most of us always find ways to rationalize why we can't or shouldn't do them. And the sad thing is, trying new things — whether it be traveling to a new place, learning a new skill, or just doing something out of our comfort zone — can actually be really, really good for us.

7 WAYS TO BE MORE OPEN TO NEW EXPERIENCES

New experiences can boost a loving relationship, whether you've been dating for long or you're married. If you're feeling a space in your relationship, or like you want to show more love to your partner, here are few ways to be more open to new experiences that could help.

1. Designate a Monthly Date

Even among your busy schedule or overload of responsibilities, you should still make time to go on a night date with your partner. This helps strengthen the relationship between the two of you. Also, if you want something different from the usual Netflix and relaxation, well, a dinner date would be a great deal as the memory would last long.

2. Expression of Appreciation

The warmth that a relationship provides is the reason why we tend to ignore what our partner does. Instead, we tend to see their kind gestures and behaviors as our rights. To be honest, your partner doesn't have to either fill your gas tank, or buy your favorite ice cream in order for you to feel grateful. You should be able to recognize their love and respect regardless – it is the recognition of such feelings that strengthen your partner's consideration.

3. Change Schedule

It's okay, you are independent and do not plan (and you shouldn't) to stop your life for anyone. While you have other obligations other than your partnership, it's a kind gesture and compares the two schedules to see whether more time can be spent together. You may have the opportunity to go to the gym before you want to participate in your film premieres, or you may be able to wake up early in order to do your projects so you can play the intra-mural game of your partner. Although you do not have to sacrifice your life to please your partner, you need to be sufficient to make your partner happy.

4. Show Affection

In addition to showing your thanks to your partner, I will also suggest acts to demonstrate your interest in them. You will know how to feel about your partner by grabbing his/her hand at a restaurant or in bed at the end of the night.

TECHNIQUE 6: CREATING A SENSE OF SECURITY IN YOUR RELATIONSHIP

It's not uncommon for both women and men to feel insecure in a relationship from time to time. We often see emotional in security as an underlying issue to address with couples who come to us for marriage counseling, couples therapy, premarital counseling and relationship coaching. After all, when couples don't feel completely emotionally safe and secure with each other it tends to create conflict and problems in many other areas of their partnership.

It's especially true for people in new relationships to have some anxiety, but even people in long-term relationships can worry about their partner's feelings forthem sometimes. While very common, feeling insecure in your relationship can create problems — for both ofyou.

ROOT CAUSES OF INSECURITY

If insecurity is an issue in your relationship — either for you, or your partner — you might be speculating about the root causes of insecurity and how to heal them. People can struggle to feel emotionally safe with their partner for a variety of reasons — sometimes due to their life experiences, but sometimes, due to things that have happened in the current relationship itself.

Insecurity After Infidelity - Certainly being let down or betrayed by your partner in the past can lead you to struggle with trust in the present moment. Insecurity after infidelity or an emotional affair is very common. In these cases, the path to healing can be a long one. The person who did the betraying often needs to work very hard, for a long time, to show (not tell, but show) their partners that they can trust them.

Anxiety After Being Let Down Repeatedly - However, insecurities can also start to emerge after less dramatic betrayals and disappointments. Even feeling that your partner has not been emotionally available for you, has not been consistently reliable, or was there for you in a time of need, it can lead you to question the strength of their commitment and love.

Trust is fragile: If your relationship has weathered storms, learning how to repair your sense of trust and security can be a vital part of healing. Often, couples need to go back into the past to discuss the emotional wounds they experienced with each other in order to truly restore the bond of safety and security. These conversations can be challenging, but necessary.

Insecurity Due to having Been Hurt in the Past - Sometimes people who have had negative experiences in past relationships can feel insecure, due to having been traumatized by others. For some people, their very first relationships were with untrustworthy or inconsistent parents and that led to the development of insecure attachment styles. This can lead them to feel apprehensive or protective with anyone who gets close. However, even people with loving parents and happy childhoods can carry scars of past relationships, particularly if they lived through a toxic relationship at some point in their lives. Its completely understandable: Having been burned by an ex can make it harder to trust a new partner, due to fears of being hurt again.

Long Distance Relationships - Certainty of relationships can lead people to feel less secure than they'd like to, simply due to the circumstances of the relationship itself. For example, you might feel more insecure if you're in a long-distance relationship. Not being able to connect with your partner or see them in person all the time can take a toll on even the strongest relationship. Couples in long-distance relationships should expect that they will have to work a little harder than couples who are together day-to-day, in order to help each person to feel secure and loved. In these cases, carefully listening to each other about what both of you are needing to feel secure and loved is vital, as is being intentionally reliable and consistent.

Feeling Insecure When you're Dating Someone New - And, as we all know, early-stage romantic love is a uniquely vulnerable experience and often fraught with anxiety. Dating someone new is exciting, but it can also be intensely anxiety-provoking. In new (or new-ish) relationships where a commitment has not been established, not fully knowing

Where you stand with a new person that you really like is emotionally intense. If you're dating, or involved in a new relationship, you may need to deliberately cultivate good self-soothing and calming skills in order to manage the emotional rollercoaster that new love can unleash.

Feeling Insecure with a Withdrawn Partner - Interestingly, different types of relationship dynamics can lead to differences in how secure people feel. The same person can feel very secure and trusting in one relationship, but with a different person, feel suspicious, worried, and on pins and needles. Often this has to do with the relational dynamic of the couple.

For example, in relationships where one person has a tendency to withdraw, be less communicative, or is not good at verbalizing their feelings it can lead their partner to feel worried about what's reallygoing on inside of them. This can turn into a pursue-withdraw dynamic that intensifies over time; one person becoming increasingly anxious and agitated about not being able to get through to their partner, and the withdrawn person clamping down like a clam under assault by a hungry seagull. However, when communication improves and couples learn how to show each other love and respect in the way they both need to feel safe and secure, trust is strengthened and emotional security is achieved.

TYPES OF INSECURITIES

Emotional security (or lack of) is complex. In addition, to having a variety of root causes, there are also different ways that insecurity manifests in people —and they all have an impact on your relationship. As has been discussed in past articles on this blog, people who struggle with low self esteem may find it hard to feel safe in relationships because they are anticipating rejection. The "insecure over achiever" may similarly struggle to feel secure in relationships if they're not getting the validation and praise they thrive on.

For others, insecurity is linked to an overall struggle with vulnerability and perfectionism. People who feel like they need to be perfect in order to beloved can — subconsciously or not — tryto hide their flaws. But, on a deep level, they know they're not perfect (no one is) and so that knowledge can lead to feelings of apprehension when they let other people get close to them. In these cases, learning how to lean into authentic vulnerability can be the path of healing.

Sometimes people who are going through a particularly hard time in other parts of their lives can start to feel apprehensive about their standing in their relationship. For example, people who aren't feeling great about their career can often feel insecure when they're around people who they perceive as being more successful or accomplished than they are. This insecurity is heightened in the case of a layoff or unexpected job loss. If one partner in a relationship is killing it, and the other is feeling under-employed or like they're still finding their way, it can lead the person who feels dissatisfied with their current level of achievement to worry that their partner is dissatisfied with them too.

Insecurities can take many forms, and emerge for a variety of reasons. However, when insecurity is running rampant the biggest toll it takes is often on a relationship.

HOW INSECURITY CAN RUIN A RELATIONSHIP

To be clear: Having feelings is 100% okay. Nothing bad is going to happen to you, or your relationship, or anyone else because you have feelings of anxiety or insecurity. The only time relationship problems occur as a result of feelings is when your feelings turn into behaviors.

If people who feel insecure, anxious, jealous or threatened don't have strategies to soothe themselves and address their feelings openly with their partner (and have those conversations lead to positive changes in the relationship), the feelings can lead to behaviors that can harm the relationship. Some people lash out in anger when they perceive themselves to be in emotional danger, or that their partner is being hurtful to them. Often, people who feeling secure will attempt to control their partner's behaviors in efforts to reduce their own anxiety. Many insecure people will hound their partners for information about the situations they feel worried about. Still others will withdraw, pre-emptively, as a way of protecting themselves from the rejection they anticipate.

While all of these strategies are adaptive when you are in a situation where hurtful things are happening, (more on toxic relationships here) problems occur when these defensive responses flareup in a neutral situation. A common example of this is the scenario where one person repeatedly asks their partner if they're cheating on them because they feel anxious, when their partner is actually 100% faithful to them and has done nothing wrong. The insecure person might question their partner, attack their partner, check up on their partner, or be cold and distant due to their worries about being cheated on or betrayed — when nothing bad is actually happening. This leaves the person on the other side feeling hurt, controlled, rejected, vilified or simply exhausted.

If feelings of insecurity are leading to problematic behaviors in a relationship, over time, if unresolved, it can erode the foundation of your partnership.

FIVE WAYS TO INCREASE SECURITY IN YOUR RELATIONSHIP

- **Do Not Try to Read Your Partner's Mind** – A common problem among couples is that they do not have deep conversations about their future, what they love and hate.
  At some point, every gesture made by any of them might be perceived in the wrong way by the other party, and moments like this should be avoided because they tend to bring fights that have no sense.
- **A Perfect Relationship Does Not Exist** - Stop looking for the perfect relationship, for the ideal man, for the perfect woman, the perfect body, or the perfect eyes. If they love you, if they are with you in good and bad times, if they bring you ice cream at 2 a.m., then you have found the perfect someone. It is always the picture in our head about how it is supposed to be that ruins every relationship that we have and makes us not see what beauty surrounds us, leading to a failure of a relationship. Everyone is perfect in their own way, you just have to go and find the small perfections in the imperfection.
- **Leave the Past at The Door** - What kind of a relationship will you have if you continually remind your boyfriend or girlfriend about every single mistake that your ex has done to hurt you? Of course, they hurt you; that is the reason why they are no longer your partner! Even if it was cheating, not paying enough attention to you, or simply breaking up with you because they did not consider that you were good enough for them, they still broke your heart.
- **Where There Is No Problem Do Not Make One Up** - If your relationship has not had any problems until now, no not try to start

finding ways of getting into stupid fights: the toilet seat is still up, the toothpaste cap is not on, the juice is too warm or your beer opener is not where it is supposed to be. Start forgiving the minor "problems" that you think your partner is making, and you never know what problems you may cause him or her! The small fights are not that important, but when they start to happen often, even daily, they may cause a rupture that no one will repair.

- **Start Focusing on The Positive Things That Are Happening to You** - We all are different, we all want different things, but if we do them together in a way that we love, then we all get to the perfect relationship easily. If you have a problem in the present, look at the future with optimism. If you had a problem in the past, look at the present with appreciation. Be grateful for every beautiful moment that you share together, and be thankful for every beautiful moment that comes to you. You will remember it with grace, whatever the future may bring.

HOW TO HELP YOUR PARTNER FEEL MORE SECURE

It's not uncommon for partners of in secure people to seek support through therapy or life coaching, or couples counseling either for themselves or with their partners. They ask, "How do I help my wife feel more secure," or "How do I help my husband feel more secure." This is a great question; too often partners put the blame and responsibility for insecure feelings squarely on the shoulders of their already-anxious spouse or partner. This, as you can imagine can only make things worse.

While creating trust in a relationship is a two-way street, taking deliberate and intentional action to help your partner feel emotionally safe with you in the ways that are most important to him or her is the cornerstone of helping your insecure girlfriend, insecure boyfriend, or insecure spouse feel confident in your love for them. The key here is consistency, and being willing to do things to help them feel emotionally secure even if you don't totally get it. This is especially true of the origins of your partner's worrystem from early experiences of being hurt or betrayed by someone else.

Tips to help your spouse feel more secure:

- Ask them what they need from you to feel emotionally safe and loved by you
- Give that to them (over and over again, without being asked every time)
- Rinse and repeat

Good communication is an important part of all relationships and is an essential part of any healthy partnership. All relationships have ups and downs, but a healthy communication style can make it easier to deal with conflict and build a stronger and healthier partnership. We often hear how important communication is, but not what it is and how we can use good communication in our relationships.

TECHNIQUE 7: COMMUNICATION IS THE KEY TO A HAPPY RELATIONSHIP

By definition, communication is the transfer of information from one place to another. In relationships, communication allows to you explain to someone else what you are experiencing and what your needs are. The act of communicating not only helps to meet your needs, but it also helps you to be connected in your relationship.

COMMUNICATING CLEARLY IN A RELATIONSHIP

Talk to each other. No matter how well you know and love each other, you cannot read your partner's mind. We need to communicate clearly to avoid misunderstandings that may cause hurt, anger, resentment or confusion.

It takes two people to have a relationship and each person has different communication needs and styles. Couples need to find a way of communicating that suits their relationship. Healthy communication styles require practice and hardwork. Communication will never be perfect all the time.

Be clear when communicating with your partner, so that your message can be received and understood. Double check your understanding of what your partner is saying.

When you talk to your partner, try to:

- Set aside time to talk without interruption from other people or distractions like phones, computers or television
- Think about what you want to say
- Be clear about what you want to communicate
- Make your message clear, so that your partner hears it accurately and understands what you mean
- Talk about what is happening and how it affects you
- Talk about what you want, need and feel – use 'I' statements such as 'I need', 'I want' and 'I feel'
- Accept responsibility for your own feelings
- Listen to your partner. Put aside your own thoughts for the time being and try to understand their intentions, feelings, needs and wants (this is called empathy)
- Share positive feelings with your partner, such as what you appreciate and admire about them, and how important they are to you
- Be aware of your tone of voice
- Negotiate and remember that you don't have to be right all the time. If the issue you are having is not that important, try to let the issue go, or agree to disagree.

Non-verbal Communication

When we communicate, we can say a lot without speaking. Our body posture, tone of voice and the expressions on our face all convey a message. These non-verbal means of communicating can tell the other person how we feel about them.

If our feelings don't fit with our words, it is often the non-verbal communication that gets 'heard' and believed. For example, saying 'I love you' to your partner in a flat, bored tone of voice, gives two very different messages. Notice whether your body language reflects what you are saying.

LISTENING AND COMMUNICATION

Listening is a very important part of effective communication. A good listener can encourage their partner to talk openly and honestly. Tips for good listening include:

- Keep comfortable eye contact (where culturally appropriate)
- Lean towards the other person and make gestures to show interest and concern
- Have an open, non-defensive, fairly relaxed posture with your arms and legs uncrossed
- Face the other person – don't sit or stand sideways
- Sit or stand on the same level to avoid looking up to or down on the other person
- Avoid distracting gestures such as fidgeting with a pen, glancing at papers, or tapping your feet or fingers
- Be aware that physical barriers, noise or interruptions will make good communication difficult. Mute telephones or other communication devices to ensure you are really listening
- Let the other person speak without interruption
- Show genuine attention and interest
- Use assertive statements like 'I feel …. About …', 'what I need is …' Be aware of your tone
- Be prepared to take time out if you are feeling really angry about something. It might be better to calm down before you address the issue
- Ask for feedback on your listening from the other person

IMPROVING COMMUNICATION IN A RELATIONSHIP

Open and clear communication can be learnt. Some people find it hard to talk and may need time and encouragement to express their views. These people may be good listeners, or they may be people whose actions speak louder than their words.

You can help to improve your communication by:

- Building companionship – sharing experiences, interests and concerns with your partner, and showing affection and appreciation.
- Sharing intimacy – intimacy is not only a sexual connection. Intimacy is created by having moments of feeling close and attached to your partner. It means being able to comfort and be comforted, and to be open and honest. An act of intimacy can be as simple as bringing your partner a cup of tea because you can tell they are tired.
- Finding one or two key issues you can agree on, such as how finances are distributed, a goal you have, or your parenting styles or strategies.

To improve the way you communicate, start by asking questions such as:

What things cause conflict between you and yourpartner? Are they because you are not listening to each other?

1. *What things bring you happiness and feelings of connection?*

2. *What things cause you disappointment and pain?*

3. *What things don't you talk about and what stops you talking about them?*

4. *How would you like your communication with your partner to be different?*

If possible, ask these questions with your partner and share your responses. Consider, and try, ways to communicate differently. See whether theresults improve your communication.

When you are more aware of how you communicate, you will be able to have more control over what happens between you. While it may not be easy at first, opening up new areas of communication can lead to a more fulfilling relationship.

Some Things Are Difficult to Communicate

Most of us find some experiences or topics difficult to talk about. It might be something that is painful or makes us feel uncomfortable. For example, some people find it difficult to express their emotions. It is often the things that cannot be talked about that hurt the most.

If you are having difficulty expressing yourself, or talking with your partner about something, you might find it helps to talk to a counsellor.

- Tips for how to manage conflict with communication include:
- Avoid using the silent treatment.
- Don't jump to conclusions. Find out all the facts rather than guessing at motives.
- Discuss what actually happened, don't judge.
- Learn to understand each other, not to defeat each other.
- Talk using the future and present tense, not the past tense.
- Concentrate on the major problem, and don't get distracted by other minor problems.
- Talk about the problems that hurt your or your partner's feelings, then move on to problems about differences in opinions.
- Use 'I feel' statements, not 'You are' statements.

Seeking Help for Communication Issues

If you can't seem to improve the communication in your relationship, consider talking with a relationship counsellor. Counsellors are trained to recognise the patterns in a couple's communication that are causing problems and to help change those patterns, as well as providing strategies, tips and a safe place to explore issues.

You could also consider doing a course that is relevant to your relationship. It is better to act early and talk to someone about your concerns, rather than wait until things get worse.

5 TIPS FOR COMMUNICATING BETTER IN YOUR RELATIONSHIP

1. Ask Open-Ended Questions

Communication is not just about talking about each other's days and saying what you had to eat for lunch. It's about being able to dig deep and get to know this person as well as you can. It's not always easy to dig deep, especially for those who have never been comfortable talking about their feelings. And it's not necessary to make every conversation a heart to heart.

There are ways to do this without pressuring your S.O. to spill their deepest secrets. For example, instead of asking yes or no questions like "Did you have a good day?" try asking more open-ended questions like, "How was your day?" Yes, they may respond with a brief non-answer ("good", "fine", "the same"), but asking open-ended questions gives them an opportunity to share more if they choose to. Keep in mind that not everyone opens up so easily. Be patient with your partner if they are not sharing all the time. We set boundaries around our emotions and everyone's boundaries are different. So, be mindful and respectful of their emotional boundaries, and they should be equally mindful and respectful of yours.

2. Pick Up on Non-verbal Cues

If your partner says "my day was fine" but their tone sounds irritated, upset, or angry, then there may be something else that they're feeling but not yet ready to communicate. Communication is not just about the words we say but also how we say them. Our tone and our attitude gives away a lot more than just the words coming out of our mouths. And it's honestly a skill to be able to pick up on those non-verbal cues. Look at your S.O.'s facial expressions, their hands (are they trembling/fidgety?), their body language (Are they making eye contact? Are they crossing their arms?) and listen to their tone of voice.

3. Don't Try to Read Their Mind

Sometimes you can tell just by looking at someone what they may be feeling. It's not always easy to do this and let's face it: as much as we want to be mind readers, we aren't and shouldn't have to be. So, if you're not sure what your partner is feeling, ask them.

If you're the one holding things in and expecting your partner to ready our mind, take a moment to appreciate the fact that your partner is making an effort by asking you what's going on rather than ignoring the problem. Do your best to let them know how you're feeling when you're ready to open up about it. It's not healthy to say you're okay when you're not and then get mad at your partner for not figuring it out. Be honest about how you feel to the best of your ability, and try to express it in a healthy way before it gets to the point where it blows up and someone says something they regret. Being direct is always better than being passive aggressive.

4. Conversations Are a Two-Way Street

As you communicate with your partner take note of how many times you say "I", "You", or "We". If the conversation is mostly about yourself, it's not really a conversation. Remember to turn it back to your S.O. and ask questions about how they feel, what their thoughts are, and what's going on with them. If you find that you're saying "You" a lot, what's the context? Are you pointing fingers and placing blame?

Relationships are about both people, and each should have an equal say about things. Both people need to feel heard and be able to share what's on their mind. If you feel like your partner is the one overtaking the conversations and you can't get a word in, it's important to let them know this. They may not be aware that they're dominating the conversation. Conversations are like a tennis match; it should flow naturally back and forth to each person.

5. Tell Them What You Need from Them

Sometimes I just want to vent and feel validated by having my partner support me by saying, "Yeah that really sucks I'm sorry!" Othertimes, I want advice. Like I said before, none of us are mind readers, so it's important to try to keep your partner informed so that you're on the same page. Saying something before hand like, "I need to vent right now and I'm not looking for any advice, just your support," or, "I really need your advice on this situation," will let them know exactly what you need in that moment.

Being direct about what you need can alleviate some of the misunderstanding or stress in a given situation, too. By letting them know ahead of time, we can prevent unnecessary disagreements created by miscommunication.

Communication Is a Skill

Ultimately, communication is a skill, which means there's always room for improvement. Work together with your partner to figure out how you can maintain healthy communication and stay on the same page. Be as honest, direct, kind, and thoughtful as you can. Whether it's with a Bae Sesh, or simply making a bigger effort to open up to each other.

All romantic relationships go through ups and downs and they all take work, commitment, and a willingness to adapt and change with your partner. But whether your relationship is just starting out or you've been together for years, there are steps you can take to build a healthy relationship. Even if you've experienced a lot of failed relationships in the past or have struggled before to rekindle the fires of romance in your current relationship, you can find ways to stay connected, find fulfillment, and enjoy lasting happiness.

TECHNIQUE 8: KEEP YOUR RELATIONSHIP FLOURISHING

Every relationship is unique and people come together for many different reasons. Part of what defines a healthy relationship is sharing a common goal for exactly what you want the relationship to be and where you want it to go and that's something you'll only know by talking deeply and honestly with your partner.

However, there are also some characteristics that most healthy relationships have in common. Knowing these basic principles can help keep your relationship meaningful, fulfilling and exciting whatever goals you're working towards or challenges you're facing together.

You maintain a meaningful emotional connection with each other. You each make the other feel loved and emotionally fulfilled. There's a difference between being loved and feeling loved. When you feel loved, it makes you feel accepted and valued by your partner, like someone truly gets you. Some relationships get stuck in peaceful coexistence, but without the partners truly relating to each other emotionally. While the union may seem stable on the surface, a lack of ongoing involvement and emotional connection serves only to add distance between two people.

You're not afraid of (respectful) disagreement. Some couples talk things out quietly, while others may raise their voices and passionately disagree. The key in a strong relationship, though, is not to be fearful of conflict. You need to feel safe to express things that bother you without fear of retaliation, and be able to resolve conflict without humiliation, degradation, or insisting on being right.

You keep outside relationships and interests alive. Despite the claims of romantic fiction or movies, no one person can meet all of your needs. In fact, expecting too much from your partner can put unhealthy pressure on a relationship. To stimulate and enrich your romantic relationship, it's important to sustain your own identity outside of the relationship, preserve connections with family and friends, and maintain your hobbies and interests.

You communicate openly and honestly. Good communication is a crucial part of any relationship. When both people know what they want from the relationship and feel comfortable expressing their needs, fears, and desires, it can increase trust and strengthen the bond between you.

Falling in Love vs. Staying in Love

For most people, falling in love usually seems to just happen. It's staying in love—or preserving that "falling in love" experience—that requires commitment and work. Given its rewards, though, it's well worth the effort. A healthy, secure romantic relationship can serve as an ongoing source of support and happiness in your life, through good times and bad, strengthening all aspects of your wellbeing. By taking steps now to preserve or rekindle your falling in love experience, you can build a meaningful relationship that lasts—even for a lifetime.

Many couples focus on their relationship only when there are specific, unavoidable problems to overcome. Once the problems have been resolved they often switch their attention back to their careers, kids, or other interests. However, romantic relationships require ongoing attention and commitment for love to flourish. As long as the health of a romantic relationship remains important to you, it is going to require your attention and effort. And identifying and fixing a small problem in your relationship now can often help prevent it from growing into a much larger one down road.

The following tips can help you to preserve that falling in love experience and keep your romantic relationship healthy.

Whether you've been dating someone awhile, currently live with a partner or are part of a long-married couple, you might be seeking ways to better the relationship you have.

Unlike holiday love stories and romantic comedies in which after one or two conflicts, all is resolved, maintaining thriving relationships takes some effort. But it doesn't have to be difficult.

With the daily grind of responsibilities and frayed nerves, its understandable why dealing with partner issues falls to the bottom of your list. Just keep up with all of life's responsibilities; work, kids, neighbors, family and friends. Its taxing and many of us are plain tired, especially during difficult times, it's easier to avoid facing your stalling relationship or eroded intimacy issues.

Surely there are a few tried-and-true methods that work to improve relationships: be a good listener, carve out time together, enjoy a quality sex life and divvy up those pesky chores.

7 WAY TO KEEP YOUR RELATIONSHIP ALIVE

While those pointer shave been proven effective by relationship experts, here are seven unexpected ways to bond and enhance your relationship that might surprise you.

1. Spend Time a Part

It sounds counter intuitive as a way to improve your relationship, but take a break from your partner. Everyone needs their own space and quality time outside a relationship. Dating and marriage counselors remind us that you deserve that breathing room.

When intimacy collapses into fusion, it is not a lack of closeness but too much closeness that impedes desire. Our need for togetherness exists alongside our need for separateness. Thus, separateness is a precondition for connection: this is the essential paradox of intimacy and sex.

Individuals need time on their own for personal growth and to maintain independence within the confinesof a relationship. While individuals flourish, the relationship itself benefits. In fact, it's key to successful marriages.

Whether that means time alone to read or take a walk in the park, do it or maybe you want to attend a workout with a friend. This is especially essential right now, as partners may be spending more time together in the home due to COVID-19.

The outcome is you'll be less triggered by your partner's bothersome habits, notice that you're more patient and feel refreshed. Your special partner has time to miss you too.

2. Go to Sleep the Same Time

Perhaps you've already read that most American adults are not getting the seven to eight hours per night of healthy sleep they need. But did you know that going to bed at different times negatively impacts you and your partner?

For a healthier relationship, make sure to head to bed at the same time. There are night owls and morning birds who live on different schedules and then there are those who work in bed while the other is watching Netflix in another room. Whatever the situation, synchronize your bed time together.

Those with mismatched sleep patterns report more conflict, less conversation and have less sex than those who go to bed together.

This doesn't give you the go-ahead to dive under the covers and scroll through your social media while you're both in bed.

51% of people who are married, living together, or in a committed relationship say they their partner is distracted by their cellphone when trying to have conversations with them.

4 in 10 people are, at least, sometimes bothered by their partner's cellphone usage frequency.

3. Be Vulnerable

Sometimes you have to dig deep to be vulnerable. "Couples may find it surprising, but if each one becomes curious about one's own blind spots, discovers them, and then is courageous enough to share that vulnerability, it can help create deeper intimacy "a blind spot doesn't necessarily mean a fault or a weakness, but rather a deeply held belief about oneself or about how a relationship is supposed to work, or how love is expressed. The belief is so deep, we don't even realize we have it, hence the term blind spot.

What is an example of blind spots in relationships? "For example, one partner might discover that their tendency to micro manage people is actually related to their fear of abandonment—controlling the schedule of a loved one as a way to never be alone.

Sharing this with a partner can be a first step to changing this pattern. This should be a loving process that builds trust, not one that causes shame."

4. Create Novel Experiences

Althoug heating your favorite pizza every saturday night and incorporating rituals in your life strengthens relationships, boredom does creep in. Therefore, you should shake things up. Pepper your routine with unpredictable date nights and moments of fun.

If adventurous dates like rock climbing or learning a new language are out of the question now, can you buy a trampoline or do something unexpected? Maybe you can find other ways to bring excitement to your relationship.

Psychologist say to focus on:

- Novelty
- Variety
- Surprise
- Surprise with Little Things

Small gestures keep the spark alive and remind your partner you are thinking about them. Happy couples are kind to one another and giving or volunteering to help out is a plus. In fact, acts of kindness are powerful and those that are unplanned tend to fuel over all well-being.

Honor your partner's love language. For example, he hugs you because he values physical touch. You'd be even happier if he cleaned up the living room or spent more time away from his desk because you value acts of service and quality time together. In relationships, learn how you can show your partner your love in a way your partner would value.

Developed by Dr. Gary Chapman, an author, and counselor, the Five Love Languages are:

- Words of Affirmation
- Quality Time
- Physical Touch
- Acts of Service
- Receiving Gifts

Ways to surprise your partner:

- Bring a mug of coffee to bed
- Volunteer to do one of the other's chores
- Send a provocative text
- Hug your sweetie
- Meet your loved one at work
- Gift your partner with chocolate
- Leave lingerie on the bed
- Make eye contact and actively listen
- Wrap up a small gift
- Pen "I love you" in lipstick on the bathroom mirror
- Leave a cute sticky note on the front door or car steering wheel

5. Fight Better

While nobody wants to argue with someone they love, disagreements are in fact healthy. It's how you fight, and if you fight fairly and constructively, that matters.

Soften the StartUp: The emphasis is on your tone and intention. Speak softly and gently. Politeness goes a long way. What's key is to speak without blame. Avoid a defensive or critical remark which can cause a conflict to escalate.

Edit What You Say: Don't blurts out every negative thought. Especially when you discuss touchy topics, remember that you love the other person and maintain respect.

Offer Repair Attempts: A repair attempt is a statement or action meant to diffuse an argument. This could be using humor, touching the other person or offering an empathetic or caring remark like, "This must be difficult for you to talk about."

You could also find common ground like saying, "Well, we have different approaches, but we both want the same thing," or offer signs of appreciation throughout difficult conversations.

Focus on the Positives: Healthy and happy marriages offer a rich climate of positivity. For every negative interaction during conflict, a stable and happy marriage has five or more positive interactions.

So, try to offer five times as many positive statements in your discussions, including your arguments and disagreements. For example, a happy couple will say "Well, we do laugh a lot" instead of "We never have any fun."

Share a Loving Story: While it might surprise you, reminiscing can help enhance your relationship. Conversations that start with "Remember when" and trek down memory lane—about your first date, your first home and the funny memories—lead both of you back to good feelings. Your partner will be reminded of why they fell in love with you in the first place.

6. Show Appreciation

Another way to repair and improve your relationship is to show appreciation for certain traits your partners possesses. Always add anecdotes to demonstrate these amazing traits.

Because high-stress levels can lead to disconnection, we tend to focus on negative stories and what your partner is not doing. If you're feeling unappreciated, appreciate others. Retrain your attention on connection and positive stories.

These surprising but impactful techniques above can help you improve your relationship. Interestingly enough research shows it's not personality or compatibility that keeps couples together. It's how a couple interacts—how they speak to each other, how they get along with each other—and if they focus on building a relationship together that creates successful relationships.

7. Create Goals Together—and Separately

"Knowing what the other person wants for the future allows you to support each other in achieving dreams."

The first step for setting goals together is to get on the same page. Start by getting honest with each other about your individual goals. Knowing what the other person wants for the future allows you to support each other in achieving dreams, both together and as individuals.

Make it a point to have goal-related meetings at least once a month to check in and support one another:

- Set aside time (maybe during dinner) to chat about goals
- Hold each other accountable and ask how the other person's projects are coming along
- Open up about challenges that are keeping you from accomplishing your goals

From there, the conversation may naturally shift to big-picture goal conversation and discussion about real-life stuff. When my husband and I have these meetings, the conversation often turns into talks about finances, family, work, passions, and all the in-between stuff that gets us out of bed in the morning.

CREATE A ROADMAP: DISCUSS THE DESTINATION AND THE PLAN FOR GETTING THERE

Once goal conversations start to become more of a norm (this can take time, especially if it's a new relationship, so be patient), a more detailed strategy for creating a life together can take shape.

"This roadmap is the route we can return to when life throws its wrenches into our plans."

A road map for my husband and me allows for a broad understanding of our individual and couple goals. With this clarity, we can see the general direction of where we're headed. This roadmap is the route we can return to when life throws its wrenches into our plans. It's the thing that keeps us on track and reminds us of our dreams.

To give you a look into our roadmap, we would both love to live in a place with more nature someday; that'sour ultimate goal. So, we're in the process of discussing where to buy property or a house, and how we can make that dream a reality. We both have entrepreneurial spirits, so we're also talking about starting a business together. Creating a business and buying property are two of the stepping stones on our roadmap. Again, these are broad, big-picture goals that we'll work towards together—and as individuals.

HAVE FUN ON THE JOURNEY; DON'T GET TOO SERIOUS

Have fun in this process of mapping out the future and there's no doubt that it can get overwhelming when developing your personal and relationship goals. Practice being in the present and enjoy the process of simply dreaming (take it from the Pisces); the future will always feel a little scary and out-of-reach.

One way to do this is to dream really big—be creative and outrageous in what you want. Allow conversations to be fluid, and get excited about each other's ideas. Try not to put the other person down or brush off ideas they bring to the table, and remove judgment about how you think their goals fit into yours. These conversations expand overtime and will most likely take on many different shapes.

"Practice grace in the discomfort that comes with pursuing dreams together, and laugh when things don't go as planned."

There will be times that one or the other person in a relationship might feel stuck in their pursuits. Create an environment that leaves room for trust in discussing growing pains. Achieving goals can be uncomfortable so work towards allowing space for that discomfort.

Whether you're in a long term relationship, or just starting out, implementing goal-oriented conversations can be crucial for a healthy and long-lasting relationship. Be proactive in laying the foundation for open, transparent, and honest conversations about goals and dreams. With grace, encourage one another to move through this life, and support one another. We're all just trying to figure out what the heck we're even doing anyway.

TECHNIQUE 9: RESOLVING YOUR DIFFERENCES

It's easy to overlook one thing in today's world of dating reality programs, smartphone applications, and romantic comedies. It's rare that we "swipe right," fall in love, and then live happily ever after. Instead, when things get tough, it's tempting to give up, say "it wouldn't have worked out anyway," and go on, rather than putting in the effort to discover how to repair a relationship.

Your relationship, on the other hand, is worth preserving.

You have a background in history. You've been through a lot as a couple — many couples endure years, if not decades before they reach this point. Your partner is the one who truly understands you, and they will be there for you in ways that no one else can.

Because you're reading about how to save your relationship, you already know the first step: you must want to save it. If you have that desire, you must learn to channel it into constructive measures that will help you mend what is broken, settle underlying tensions, and salvage your relationship.

When you're in a fight with your partner, you may feel attacked or threatened, defenseless and weak, which causes you to withdraw and retreat.

When your partner disturbs you, and you feel under siege, you're less likely to act constructively and more prone to fall back on old tricks like "the silent treatment," which end up doing more harm than good. Your relationship will eventually fall apart as a result of this.

You'd almost surely respond no if someone asked you if you knew how to handle disagreement, and yes if they asked you if the silent treatment was an excellent method to deal with conflict. You know better than to use such clumsy tactics, but if you're in enough pain, you'll do it anyway. What is the reason for this?

Why revert to old habits rather than attempting to resolve the communication problems at hand?

CHECK YOUR FOCUS

When you focus on defending yourself from assault rather than tackling the problem, a confrontation becomes detrimental. If you focus on your pain and suffering, you'll get more of the same, since energy flows where focus goes, or, as Tony puts it, "whatever we persistently focus on is exactly what we will experience in our lives."

Tony used to drive on a two-lane highway with only power line posts every 10–20 yards. Flowers, candles, and photographs seemed to be adorning one of these all the time.

With so much room on either side of the post, it was incredible how many people had died or been hurt when they collided with it. So why didn't the victim manage to avoid it? Why didn't they swerve to one side or the other?

It's because people would be entirely focused on avoiding colliding with the pole. Our emphasis, on the other hand, sets our course. If we don't want to hit the pole, we must concentrate on what we want: staying on the road! So we can alter the outcome by shifting our emphasis.

This is a lesson on how to save a relationship.

Suppose you quarrel and let your anger build up instead of focusing on where you don't want your relationship to go. In that case, you'll wind up where you don't want to be — either in a miserable, unfulfilling relationship or divorced from your spouse entirely. On the other hand, you'll obtain the results you want if you focus on resolving disagreements and growing together.

TALK TO ONE ANOTHER

In a coffee shop, you're seated. Two couples are sitting beside you in the shop. The couple to your left is debating whether or not to go out to dinner with their pals. "It's never fun — you stated so yourself the previous time," he says. "Of course you'd say that," she responds, "since they're my friends, and you've never given any of my friends a chance." "Here we go," he adds sarcastically as he rolls his eyes. Our personal edition of War and Peace, book whatever." They sat silently, turning away from one other.

 The couple to your right is debating whether or not to go out to dinner with their pals. "I guess I'm a little scared that it'll go on for hours and hours and "How do you feel about it?" "I got it," she says. I really want to go, but as a compromise, can we set a time when we have to leave?" "Besides, it will be wonderful to be home early," she adds, stroking his hand and smiling. They continue to read and drink their coffee as he smiles and nods.

An issue was provided to both couples — the identical dilemma, in fact. However, one knew how to resolve interpersonal problems while the other did not. One reacted by falling back on old patterns and exploiting the issue to increase their divide. The other took advantage of the conflict to express their sentiments and strengthen their bond. Which couple do you believe has the more fulfilling and successful relationship? Which one do you think will last the longest? When it comes to saving a relationship, communication is at the top of the list.

MAKE OPPORTUNITY OUT OF CONFLICT

One couple, for example, has discovered how to resolve disputes in their relationship by going to a coffee shop: Don't be defensive, don't drive home your point, and don't attempt to win. Why would you want to lose your lover, the person you adore? You can let go of petty fights and embrace healthy communication once you recognize that there are no losers in love.

Conflicts provide you and your partner the chance to align your values and goals. In addition, they provide opportunities to learn about, appreciate, and embrace differences.Put yourself in your partner's shoes and try to comprehend what he or she is going through. These feelings and experiences may be unpleasant, but we will never grow if we consistently choose comfort over growth.

Conflict provides an opportunity to learn more about your mate and to love them even more deeply. Instead of seeing disputes as causes to retreat, learn to see them as opportunities to grow. Choose to see the great in the circumstance rather than the negative, and actively decide to work toward a more solid future together the next time you dispute with your partner and question how to save your relationship.

ASK APPROPRIATE QUESTIONS

If you're looking for ways to save a relationship, things have likely been going wrong for a while. So you must go back in time to identify the genuine, deeper concerns, and forward in time. It's all about posing the right questions to yourself. First and foremost, make sure you're in the appropriate frame of mind when you begin this practice. The goal isn't to assign blame, rehash prior disputes, or tell your partner about all the things that irritate you. Instead, you must adopt an attitude of thankfulness and acceptance. Accept the fact that life is occurring for you rather than to you. Even the current status of your relationship is an opportunity for you to grow.

PRACTICE FORGIVENESS

You're probably furious, bitter, hurt, mistrustful, and a whole host of other unpleasant emotions if you're asking how to salvage your relationship after your trust was violated. If you're the one who betrayed the trust, you're probably feeling guilty and embarrassed. You can even try to blame or justify your behaviors on your partner. Both couples must work on forgiveness in this case.

You won't suddenly feel forgiving toward your lover when you wake up one day. Forgiveness is a process that takes time. It's a succession of tiny gestures over time — admitting mistakes, exercising complete honesty, and prioritizing your spouse. It takes effort to forgive.

If you were the one who betrayed your partner's trust, you must accept full responsibility. Respect your partner's feelings and offer them the space they require. Avoid falling into a cycle of self-blame by prioritizing your relationship. If your trust has been damaged, give yourself some space while continuing to communicate. Tell your partner what you need in order to re-establish trust. Never ever give up.

Relationships are difficult. We are all human beings, and we make mistakes. We are not without flaws. We don't always put in the effort we need to, and our relationships suffer as a result. Often we start thinking about saving a relationship after ignoring it for years. However, keep in mind that many relationships are worth preserving. All you have to do is be willing to put in the effort.

CHAPTER 6: LONGING FOR CONNECTIONS

Albert Camus once stated that, "in order to understand the world, one has to turn away from it on occasion."

What one can understand from this is that solitude gives us the space we need to contemplate the world we experience. It's a private time especially for us to go over our day, as well as our reactions to it. Our emotions, thoughts, worries, desires... They all become clearer to us when we scrutinize them in the light of ourselves. Yet despite this, most of us equate solitude with loneliness and therefore it brings about misery. Recent studies claim that three out of four people suffer from "loneliness". Countries the world over have declared that there's an epidemic of loneliness, though that's not necessarily the case. In fact, what we suffer from might not be loneliness but It might just be our inability to understand and embrace solitude and therefore ourselves.

Running Away From Ourselves to Escape Loneliness

Simply defined loneliness is the longing for human connection. It's being unable to form a true connection with others when we're surrounded by others, and similarly being unable to connect with ourselves when we're alone. This can leave us feeling lonely, for example, when we're home or out alone, despite being with ourselves or even surrounded by others. We've become so disconnected that we think we're lonely when we don't have anyone other than ourselves to talk to.

If we want to form genuine connections and if we want to be rid of our loneliness and restlessness, then we must first change our relationship and understanding of "solitude". We must redefine what being alone means for us, along with our relationship with ourselves. Only then can we begin to form true connections with others.

We all experience difficult emotions sometimes: Anger, fear, loneliness... These emotions are remnants of the survival mechanisms that kept us alive during the stone age. We feel fear because it allows us to run from danger, we feel anger because it propels us to fight an enemy, and loneliness works almost the same way.

Consider this: why are we able to feel lonely? Why do we have the need to connect with others? Humans has survived for hundreds of years by banding together. To quote Game of Thrones: "When winter comes, the lone wolf dies but the pack survives." So to survive winter and other difficult situations, we need one another. We need a tribe, family, friends... In the past human beings used to live in tribes of 150-200 people.

Everyone in the tribe knew and supported each other, because they needed and depended on one another. They had actual conversations because ephemeral ones would never serve them. They shared information, experiences, thoughts, feelings... They imparted what they learned to the generations that came after them. Driven by their needs, they formed actual communities and relationships. So what happened between then and now?

We still have an innate need to connect with others. But when we lack that connection with others, loneliness begins to creep in. But imagine if we couldn't feel lonely. Imagine that "loneliness" did not exist. If that were the case, would you ever feel the need or desire to go out of your house and hang out with people? Would you seek either friendships or relationships? Of course, not. So, in a weird way, loneliness prompt us to get up, walk away from the TV and seek human connection. Our ability to feel lonely is to a degree responsible for our families, love lives and friendships. That is, as long as we are able to properly define loneliness and our relationship to it.

If we're lucky – and most of us are luckier than we think – we'll form bonds with people who will appreciate the trust and confidence we have in them. Not only that, they'll reciprocate it. That is to say, they will trust us with parts of themselves as well. They will acknowledge the risk we're taking in trusting them little by little and also begin to approach us with more about themselves. Over time, if that mutual trust is respected and preserved, it will grow over time and develop into a dependable and strong connection. This type of connection gives us as humans a great deal of comfort, support and resilience. In a sense it translates as, "I see who you are. This is who I am and I am here for you".

TECHNIQUE 10: MAKE NEW FRIENDS

Why are friends so important?

Our society tends to place an emphasis on romantic relationships. We think that just finding that right person will make us happy and fulfilled. But research shows that friends are actually even more important to our psychological welfare. Friends bring more happiness into our lives than virtually anything else.

Friendships have huge impact on your mental health and happiness. Good friends relieve stress, provide comfort and joy, and prevent loneliness and isolation. Developing close friendships can also have a powerful impact on your physical health. Lack of social connection may pose much of a risk as smoking, drinking too much, or leading a sedentary lifestyle. Friend's are even tied to longevity. One Swedish study found that, along with physical activity, maintaining a rich network of friends can add significant years to your life.

But close friendships don't just happen. Many of us struggle to meet people and develop quality connections. Whatever your age or circumstances, though, it's never too late to make new friends, reconnect with old ones, and greatly improve your social life, emotional health, andoverall well-being.

The Benefits of Friendships

While developing and maintaining friendships takes time and effort, healthy friendships can:

Improve Your Mood - Spending time with happy and positive friends can elevate your mood and boost your outlook.

Help You to Reach Your Goals - Whether you're trying to get fit, give up smoking, or otherwise improve your life, encouragement from a friend can really boost your will power and increase your chances of success.

Reduce Your Stress and Depression - Having an active social life can bolster your immune system and help reduce isolation, a major contributing factor to depression.

Support You Through Tough Times - Even if it's just having someone to share your problems with, friends can help you cope with serious illness, the loss of a job or loved one, the breakup of a relationship, or any other challenges in life.

Support You as You Age - As you age, retirement, illness, and the death of loved ones can often leave you isolated. Knowing there are people you can turn to for company and support can provide purpose as you age and serve as a buffer against depression, disability, hardship and loss.

Boost Your Self-Wort - Friendship is a two-way street and the "give" side of the give-and-take contributes to your own sense of self-worth. Being there for your friends make you feel needed and adds purpose to your life.

WHAT TO LOOK FOR IN A FRIEND?

A friend is someone you trust and with whom you share a deep level of understanding and communication. A good friend will:

- Show a genuine interest in what's going on in your life, what you have to say, and how you think and feel.

- Accept you for who you are.
- Listen to you attentively without judging you, telling you how to think or feel, or try changing the subject.
- Feel comfortable sharing things about themselves with you.

As friendship works both ways, a friend is also someone you feel comfortable supporting and accepting, and someone with whom you share a bond of trust and loyalty.

Focus on the way friendship feel, not what it looks like.

The most important quality in a friendship is the way the relationship makes you feel—not how it looks on paper, how alike you seem on the surface, or what others think. Ask yourself:

- *Do I feel better after spending time with this person?*
- *Am I around this person?*
- *Do I feel secure, or do I feel like I have to watch what I say and do?*
- *Is the person supportive and am I treated with respect?*
- *Is this a person I can trust?*

The bottomline: if the friendship feels good, it is good. But if a person tries to control you, criticizes you, abuses your generosity, or brings unwanted drama or negative influences into your life, it's time to re-evaluate the friendship. For example, a good friend does not require you to compromise your values, always agree with them, or disregard your own needs.

Evaluating Interest

Friendship takes two, so it's important to evaluate whether the other person is looking for new friends.

- *Do they ask your personal questions, as if they'd like to get to know you better?*
- *Do they tell you things about themselves beyond surface small talk?*
- *Do they give you their full attention when you see them?*

- *Does the other person seem interested in exchanging contact information or making specific plans to get together?*

If you can't answer "yes" to these questions, the person may not be the best candidate for friendship now, even if they genuinely like you. There are many possible reasons why not, so don't take it personally!

HOW TO MAKE NEW FRIENDS: WHERE TO START

We tend to make friends with people we cross paths with regularly: people we go to school with, work with, or live close to. The more we see someone, the more likely we develop friendship. So, look at the places you frequent as you start your search for potential friends.

Another big factor in friendship is common interests. We tend to be drawn to people who are similar, with a shared hobby, cultural background, career path, or kids the same age. Think about activities you enjoy or the things you care about and you wonder where you can meet people who share the same interests.

No matter what's happening in your life, you will want friends by your side! With the rise of technology, making friends online is a growing and common occurrence. This is especially true and it's useful if you are someone who is attending online college. That's why knowing how to make friends online can have a tremendous and positive impact your experience while at an online college, and in general in your life.

When you attend a traditional on-campus school, you will make friends in class, study halls, and at on-campus events. But when you attend an online college, you will need to try new methods to build friendships.

Here are some helpful tips on where and how to establish, grow, and maintain online friendships.

Messaging Friends Online in a Chat

Finding friends online goes hand-in-hand with finding new friends in real life. It still requires that you take part in activities within your community and can evolve said friendships online.

176

Some places where you can expect to find new friends both in person and online include:

1. Study groups: Create or join a group for students at your college. Then you can offer to meet for study groups or join already existing study groups.

2. Do things you love in your city: One of the best ways to make friends is to take part in activities you enjoy. That way, you can meet people with similar interests with whom you can continue the activity. You can leverage online websites to find events you're interested in, whether that be through social media or checking a gym's schedule of classes online, for example.

3. Join a group online based on your likes: Based on your interest's and hobbies, try to perform a search online to find a group that shares in your hobby. Then, connect online and set up in-person meetings to perform the interest. For example, you can find people who like to paint online and then setup a wine and paint night!

4. Connect on social media: From Facebook to Instagram, and Snapchat to Twitter, there are plenty of social media platforms where you can make new friends.

Start a Conversation Online and Next Steps

Once you locate the digital places where you can connect with like-minded and potential friends, the next step is saying hello and making plans. This is where a lot of people struggle because connecting online can feel less personal.

People don't want to come off as weird or creepy online, so here are some tips on how to start the conversation:

1. Start a conversation that leads to meeting up: When you join a social media group or group online, start to be active in the group. Like and comment onother people's posts and then consider posting and sharing yourself. People will start to recognize your name as you recognize theirs. Some people may reach out first, but if not, you can at least begin to build a connection through consistent communication. Then you can take the next step to send a personal message.

2. Send a message to someone you want to get to know: Once you decide who you want to be friend, send a message! You can reach out by sharing something you related to that they shared and ask a question, or just share your support for something they've shared, then let the conversation unfold naturally.

3. Ask questions to continue conversations: A goodway to keep a conversation going is to ask questions. Most people who want to engage in conversation will ask questions back if they are interested. This will give you a sign to know if there's something worth growing with them.

Are Online Friendships Meaningful as In-Person Relationships?

The main components of friendship include: freedom to choose, intimacy, and commitment. Online friendships maintain these three things; you have the choice to become friends with or end friendships with whomever you wish, Secondly, you are able to be intimate through what you choose to share with one another and, lastly, you can continue your commitment to the friendship by communicating over time.

Keep Your Options Open

When it comes to choosing friends online and using applications, you should narrow down your search to be very specific. You may see things you aren't looking for and swipe left instead of right on what could potentially have become your next best friend. Sometimes, it pays to keep an open mind when online friendship matching. This is because it can mirror your experience like real life.

Think of this: when you go out in public places, you never know who you will meet. The randomness of new connections is sometimes what makes the mall more worthwhile. As such, you should practice the same open-minded attitude when meeting people online in that way, you can expand your opportunities to meet new people. Only once you get to know them better can you truly assess whether or not it is a relationship worth pursuing or not.

Build Your Self-Confidence - Liking yourself before going off in search of friends is an important step to take in building healthy relationships.

"Think about what you like about yourself when you're comfortable with yourself, it shines out of you."

Find Something You Feel Passionate About - Join a language class if you love languages or volunteer outdoors if you love nature. "That's where you'll find friendships."

Put Yourself out There - Remember, nothing ventured, and nothing gained. "It isn't that you lose if you meet someone and it doesn't fit for a friendship, that's not losing, that's having tried."

Meet in a Neutral Place - Once you have taken the first step and are moving on to meeting outside the initial environment where you made a connection, chose a neutral public space. This can lessen the pressures that, say, hosting at home can bring, and give you time to focus on each other.

Ask Questions - If you want to be popular, ask people about themselves and listen sincerely when they answer. A good listener is rare these days, It is the best passport you could possibly have to friendship.

Don't Expect too Much - A common mistake is expecting too much from one person. It is more realistic and healthier to have a variety of friends for different reasons.

TECHNIQUE 11: GET SUPPORT FROM YOUR OTHER-HALF

Dating someone with anxiety issues or an anxiety disorder can be horribly stressful. Sometimes it can feel like the anxiety is a third person in the relationship, someone who wriggles between you and your partner. This person constantly sow doubt and confusion.

No one prepared you for this, and you can't choose who you fall for. There's no high school class on dating, muchless dating someone with a mental health condition.

Nonetheless, anxiety doesn't have to break your relationship or put a strain on it to the point where it's hard to enjoy. By understanding anxiety in general and how it affects both your partner and your relationship, you can love each other more deeply and connect in a new way. Educating yourself can also relieve a lot of the stress.

The Anxiety Coming out Conversation

Whether you ask or deduce it after months of dating, there will be a point when you partner discloses they deal with anxiety. It's a crucial moment in the relationship, so be sensitive and do not judge. Thank them for trusting you with this information that they have most likely not shared with many people. See it as the beginning of a discussion you can resurface occasionally.

Understanding Anxiety and What It is Doing to Your Partner?

- Anxiety is a real problem, not something made up. It is a mental health issue.
- Anxiety is normal. Everyone has it. It only becomes an issue or disorder if it is severe.
- Anxiety can be a debilitating illness that prevents people from functioning and living a normal life.
- Anxiety makes people experience fight-or-flight reactions and stress to issues that are not life-threatening, including worrying about whether a partner will cheat or leave.
- You cannot "fix" or "cure" anxiety.
- Most people who have anxiety wish they didn't have it. They worry about their anxiety being a burden to others.
- There are millions of people who, despite dealing with anxiety, have great relationships and arehappy.
- Symptoms of anxiety can occur in waves, consistently or both. People with anxiety disorders or issues can have periods of time when they don't experience symptoms.
- Anxiety is not logical or rational. It causes people to worry about something despite there being no evidence to suggest it is worth worrying about. It also causes them to sometimes act irrationally. Your partner most likely knows this.

- Anxiety is not a weakness.
- Anxiety is treatable. Psychotherapy can relieve symptoms and teach people how to better cope with it.

5 WAYS TO COPE WITH IT

Anxiety doesn't have to put your relationship in jeopardy. By using the right coping strategies, you can have a healthy relationship and stop anxiety from causing too much stress.

1. Encouraging Your Partner to Work with a Therapist or Try Couples Therapy

When you care for someone, it's tempting to support them by trying to pick the role of a surrogate therapist. The problem is you're not a therapist. Trying to play that role will be emotionally draining. It could make you resent your partner.

You are not responsible for providing therapy to your partner and this is why you should gently guide your partner toward working with a therapist. A therapist can help them improve how they deal with anxiety, in and outside a relationship.

So if you're in a serious, long-term relationship, consider couple's counseling, some of the anxiety issues might be based in your relationship.

Working with a couple's counselor should take the pressure off your partner. Rather than encouraging them to do something on their own, you are inviting them to join you in therapy.

What happens in couples counseling?

In couples counseling, you and your partner will gain insight into your relationship, learn how to effectively resolve conflicts, and improve your overall relationship satisfaction through various therapeutic techniques. Therapists will often assign tasks to the couple so that they can apply the skills learnt in therapy in their daily interactions. Most couples conclude therapy with a better understanding of their relational pattern sand heightened communication skills, allowing them to continue their relationship in a much healthier, more fulfilling way.

2. Going to Therapy Yourself

Whether your partner accepts or resists your suggestion to go to therapy, you should do it yourself. It will help you develop the skills necessary to understand and cope with your partner's anxiety. A therapist can also teach you how to be more effectively support your anxious partner.

When you are dating someone with anxiety, its easy to forget about taking care of yourself. By going to therapy, you can ensure you are still focusing on your own mental health.

3. Learning How to Better Communicate About the Anxiety

Anxiety can be scary. It can make you want to avoid talking about it.

Nonetheless, one of the most effective ways to cope with anxiety in a relationship is to talk about it openly, honestly and directly with your partner.

"Having can did talks together on what they are feeling and validating those feelings is paramount,"

To show your partner you accept their anxiety, you need to encourage them to open up about it. Try to listen without judging, becoming defensive or taking their anxiety personally.

4. Managing Your Reactions to the Anxiety

When your partner talks about his or her anxiety in the context of your relationship, it's easy to take it personally and become upset. It's easy to interpret the anxiety as selfishness, rejection or an attempt to create distance.

"You will want them to just get over it" - "You will want them to just not worry about it."

By practicing your coping skills, you can over ride this counter productive default response into something more compassionate. Here is a scenario to help you practice:

Imagine your partner says she has anxiety about you cheating. If you take it personally, you might think she has this anxiety because she judges you or thinks you are the kind of person who is likely to cheat.

The moment you make it about you, you'll start to feel upset. You might react defensively and say something mean.

"If you can't bend without shaming, you will only make the problem worse," Then you partner will strike back. Flash forward to an hour later and you're fighting. The argument has snow balled. You might not even remember why you are fighting.

Instead of allowing the anxiety to rile you up, take a moment to calm down. Remind yourself that the anxiety most likely isn't about you. You're not the source of it, its about your partner.

Calmly address what your partner is feeling. You can say something like, "I'm really sorry you feel that way, that must be hard. Is there anything we can do to help you feel better about that?"

Managing your reactions is more important than managing your partner's reactions, It can help you be there for your partner and set boundaries. If your partner's anxiety causes you to flip out every time they bring it up, it will be impossible to support them.

5. Setting Boundaries

When you are dating someone with anxiety, you need to strike a balance between being patient and setting boundaries. Once you recognize how their anxiety influences their behavior, you can cut them slack for behaviors you might not normally have much patience for.

Nonetheless, there should be limits to this. Even severe mental illnesses do not give people a license to be cruel or hurtful.

Don't always be the one who bends If you always yield to your partner's anxiety, you will become resentful and bitter, not towards the anxiety but toward your partner."

Here are some examples of boundaries you can set. You can tell your partner these behaviors are not acceptable, even during anxiety attacks and stressful times that cause intense anxiety:

- Insults
- Accusations
- Threats

HOW TO SUPPORT YOUR PARTNER

There's a difference between providing support and becoming your partner's unpaid, unofficial therapist. A therapist isn't going to hold your partner while they cry or take the mouth for something to help relieve the anxiety.

Acknowledge Their Progress on Anxiety Issues

If your partner is taking steps to work on anxiety, remember to acknowledge that. Always Listen!

Even if you are tired or feel like your partner is saying something you have already heard, try to listen carefully. It helps them know you care.

Include Your Partner in Self-Care/Mental Health Rituals

Do you have any rituals or hobbies you use to take care of your mental health? Maybe you meditate, run or listen to relaxing music. If so, try to include your partner.

Including your partner in rituals like this can help both of you reduce anxiety in the relationship.

What NOT to Do

To avoid making the anxiety worse, hurting your partner and creating more stress in the relationship, DO NOT:

- Criticize them for having anxiety
- Dismiss their anxiety
- Enable maladaptive anxious behaviors by coddling them too much
- Try to be their therapist

- Take everything personally
- Lose your temper or patience everytime the anxiety flares up
- Try to "fix" your partner
- Recommend drugs for their anxiety (you are not a psychiatrist)

Anxiety Can Actually Deepen Your Relationship

Anxiety isn't only a source of stress in a relationship. It's also an opportunity to understand and love your partner more deeply. The beliefs behind their anxiety is a part of who they are.

By learning about anxiety or seeking help from a mental health professional, you can support your partner and look out for your own mental health. Then your relationship can become stronger and more full of joy.

If you're someone who struggles with anxiety, there are plenty of things about you that would make loving you easy. All relationships struggle sometimes and when anxiety is at play, the struggles can be quite specific – very normal, and specific.

Anxiety can work in curious ways and it will impact different relationships differently, so not all of the following will be relevant for every relationship. Here are some ways to strengthen your relationship and protect it from the impact of anxiety:

Top up the Emotional Resources

You're probably super sensitive to the needs of others and give openly and abundantly to your relationship. Sometimes though, anxiety can drain those resources from the relationship just as quickly as you invest them. This is completely okay – there is plenty of good that comes with loving you to make up for this – but it may mean that you have to keep making sure those resources are topped up. Whenever you can, heap your partner with attention, gratitude, affection, touch – lots of touch – and conversation around him or her.

Let Your Partner See You as a Support too

Your partner might feel reluctant to 'burden' you with worries, particularly if those worries don't seem as big as the ones you're struggling with. People with anxiety have so much strength – it's impossible to live with anxiety without it – so make sure your partner knows that it doesn't matter how big or small their struggles are, you can be the supportive one sometimes too. The tendency can be for partners of anxious people to dismiss their own worries, but this might mean that they do themselves out of the opportunity to feel nurtured and supported by you – which would be a huge loss for both of you. Be deliberate in being the rock sometimes too. Ask, hold, touch. There's nothing more healing than the warmth of the person you love.

Let Your Partner in on What You're Thinking

Anxious thoughts are supremely personal, but let your partner in on them. It's an important part of intimacy. You will often be thinking about what you need to do to feel safe, what feels bad for you and what could go wrong. You will also have an enormous capacity to think of other people – anxious people do – but make sure that you let you partner in on the thoughts that arrest you. Keeping things too much to yourself have a way of widening the distance between two people.

Asking for reassurance is absolutely okay – but just not too much.

Anxiety has a way of creeping into everything. When it's left unchecked, it can make you doubt the things that don't deserve to be doubted; such as your relationship. It's completely okay and very normal to ask your partner for reassurance. Too much though and it could be felt as neediness. Neediness is the enemy of desire and overtime can smother the spark. Make sure your partner has the opportunity to love you spontaneously, without prompting – it's lovely for them and even better for you.

Be Vulnerable

Anxiety can affect relationships in different ways. In some people, it might stoke the need for constant reassurance. In others, it can cause them to hold back, to lessen their vulnerability to possible heartache.

Vulnerability – being open to another – is beautiful and it's the essence of successful, healthy relationships. The problem with protecting yourself too much is that it can invite the very rejection you're trying to protect against. Part of intimacy is letting someone in closer than you let the rest of the world. It's trusting that person with the fragile, messy, untamed parts of you; the parts that are often beautiful, sometimes baffling, and always okay with the person who loves you. It's understandable to worry about what might happen if someone has open access to these parts of you, but see those worries for what they are – worries, not realities – and trust that whatever happens when you open yourself up to loving and being loved, you'll be okay. Because you will be.

Be Careful of Projecting Anxiety onto Your Relationship

Anxiety can be triggered by nothing in particular – that's one of the awful things about it – so it will look for a target, an anchor to hold it still and make it make sense. If you're in an intimate relationship, that's where the bull's eye will sit, drawing your anxiety into its gravitational pull. This can raise feelings of doubt, jealousy, suspicion and insecurity. Anxiety can be a rogue like that. That doesn't mean your relationship deserves your anxiety – most likely it doesn't – but your relationship is important, relevant and often in your thoughts, making it lavishly an easy target. Remind yourself that just because you're worried, that doesn't mean there's anything to worry about. Worry if you have to, but then see it for what it is – anxiety, not truth. You are loved and you have anxiety and you are okay, let that be the truth that holds you.

Analysis Leads to Paralysis

There's a saying – 'Analysis leads to paralysis,' – because it does. Is it love? Or lust? Or am I kidding myself? What if my heart gets broken into tiny jagged pieces? How will it ever work if we don't like the same music/ books/ food/ movies? What if we book the holiday and the airline goes on strike? What if one of us gets sick? What if we both get sick? What if we can't get a refund? pay the mortgage? What if he gets sick of me?' Yes, I know you know how it sounds. What you focus on is what becomes important, so if you focus on the possible problems they'll absorb your energy until they're big enough to cause trouble on their own. They'll drain your energy, your sense of fun and your capacity to move. You probably already know this, but what can be done about it? Here's something to try … Set a time frame in which you can act as thoughthings will be fine. So for example, worry from 10-3 each day and after that, breathe, let go and act as though things will be fine. You don't have to believe it, just "act as though". You'll have another chance tomorrow to worry if you need to. Be guided by the evidence, not the worries that haunt you at 2am.

Understand that Your Partner Will Need Boundaries

For the relationship to stay close, healthy and connected, boundaries built by your partner can be a great thing. Understand that boundaries aren't your partner's way of keeping you out, but as a way to self-protect from 'catching' your anxiety. You might be worried and need to talk about something over and over, but that's not necessarily what will be good for you, your partner or your relationship. Your partner can love you and draw a bold heavy underline between the last time you discuss something and the next time you want to. Talking is healthy, but talking over and over and over about the same thing can be draining and create an issue where there isn't one. Know that your partner loves you and that boundaries are important to nurture love and grow the relationship, not to push against it. Talk to your partner about what he or she needs to be able to feel okay in the face of your anxiety. Invite the boundaries – it will help to keep your connection strong and loving and will help your partner to feel as though he or she is able to preserve a sense of self without being absorbed by your worries. Worry is contagious so if your partner wants to draw a boundary (eventually) around your worry, let it happen – it will help to preserve the emotional resources of the relationship and will be good for both of you.

Laugh Together

This is so important! Laughter is a natural antidote to the stress and tension that comes with anxiety. Laughing together will tighten the connection between you and when there has been a stressful few days (weeks? months?) it will help you both to remember why you fell in love with each other. Anxiety has a way of making you forget that life wasn't meant to be taken seriously all the time. If it's been too long since your partner has seen the shape of your face when you laugh (which will be beautiful and probably one of the reason she or he fell for you in the first place) find a reason – a funny movie, memories, YouTube … anything.

Falling in love is meant to be magical, but getting close to another person isn't without it's highs and low sat the best of times. From the ecstasy of realising that someone pretty wonderful is as moved by you as you are by them, to the agony of self-doubt and possible loss, to the security, richness and sometimes stillness of a deeper love, intimacy is a vehicle for every possible emotion. Anxiety does effect relationships, but by being open to its impact, and deliberate in responding to it, you can protect your relationship and make it one that's

THE EASIEST WAYS TO BE A MORE SUPPORTIVE PARTNER

Being a supportive partner can mean a lot of different things. Some of it will depend on your partner, but everyone needs support. First, there's this big picture: the big life decision type of support. "One way to become a better partner is by supporting your partner's dreams," relationship counselor Crystal Bradshaw tells Bustle. "Don't know what they are? Don't have a clue if your partner has any? Then you should ask, because this is super important stuff. I'm constantly surprised by my couples when I ask them about their life dreams, values, goals, and hopes. Often times, people tell me "I don't know what my dream is." It's partially your job to help your partner discover keep those goals and dreams alive.

In order to be a supportive partner, a lot of it comes down to the day-to-day. If you're laying the groundwork, they'll know the support is there, and you'll be in a strong position for when times get harder.

CONCLUSION

I hope this book helped you identify your anxiety issues. You learned how to solve them, identify your attachment style, and understand how jealousy and pain affect your relationship greatly.

As I stated in the introduction, I wrote this book to be used in three ways:

1. For clinicians to integrate cognitive behavioral strategies into their treatment of couples;
2. For couples to use in coordination with the work they do with their own couple therapist;
3. For couples who want to work on their own to make their relationships healthy and happy.

Throughout the course of this book, I have tried to communicate the process and strategies I use to treat couples in as straightforward, nontechnical language as I could. So, dear, I hope that you have found what I have presented in this book useful in your practice. I know I do with couple after couple, in session after session. And I am absolutely certain, dear couple, that, by mindfully and purposely putting into practice what you have learned in this book, you have moved much closer to the happy, harmonious relationship you want. Now it's time to celebrate. You've done a wonderful job. Pop open the champagne. Ring the bells. Light the fireworks.

Take a moment to consider the various emotional burdens that hold you down and keep you from feeling happy. Maybe you have a job you dislike but since you need the money to pay bills, you keep going to work there anyway, despite the fact that the atmosphere is killing your spirit. Perhaps you are in a relationship that is full of strife and arguments, as well as criticism and blame.

You need to use the lessons that I presented to you in your current relationships, rather than discarding them with the belief that doing so will resolve your anxious and unhappy feelings, because otherwise that same lesson will just pop up again in the next relationship.

When you are beset by anxiety and worry, it can feel that your thoughts control your feelings and you are helpless to change anything at all. But when you take a chance on opening your heart to others in your life and let them know you would like to be closer to them and support them in their goals, you will probably discover that they would like the same thing as well but didn't know how to break through the pattern of interaction that has become a repetitious cycle with you two.

Now, let go of the anxious feelings inside and congratulate yourself for having the maturity and strength to stop destructive behavior. Enjoy your freedom, and celebrate your new lease on life!

Take the attachment test to help you understand how to love your partner and what kind of love you require from your partner.

This book has been structured in a way that makes it easy for you to follow through each - revive the relationship and take it to a higher stage.

THANK YOU

Thank you very much for taking the time to read this book. I hope it positively impacts your life in ways you can't even imagine.

If you have a minute to spare, I would really appreciate a few words on the site where you bought it.

Honest feedbacks help readers find the right book for their needs!

A. Marie Smith

PERFECTBOUND2.0

Published by Perfect Bound 2.0 Design and Writing © 2021 Perfect Bound 2.0

9 781802 850581